# Predicting Dangerousness

# Predicting Dangerousness

## The Social Construction of Psychiatric Reality

**Stephen J. Pfohl**
Boston College

**Lexington Books**
D.C. Heath and Company
Lexington, Massachusetts
Toronto

**Library of Congress Cataloging in Publication Data**

Pfohl, Stephen J.
    Predicting dangerousness.

    Bibliography: p. 233
    Includes indexes.
    1. Violence.  2. Mental illness—Diagnosis—Social aspects.  3. Criminal
behavior, Prediction of.  4. Psychiatry—Philosophy.  I. Title.
RC569.5.V55P44                      616.8'582                      77-25742
ISBN 0-669-01509-1

Published simultaneously in Canada

Printed in the United States of America

International Standard Book Number: 0-669-01509-1

Library of Congress Catalog Card Number: 77-25742

*To my parents, family, and friends,*
*who have introduced me*
*to so many versions*
*of social reality*

# Contents

# List of Tables

# Preface

This book tells a story of professional experts at work. Yet, it is a particular kind of story—a sociological story. It attends to those things that people (in this case, psychiatric professionals) do together, do in each other's company, and do in anticipation of the doings of others. It also attends to what emerges from all of these doings—socially structured senses of reality (in this case, the reality of whether another person is or is not dangerous and/or mentally disturbed).

The story being told here, however, is not simply a sociologist's story about the work of professionals in other disciplines. Although it raises certain critical questions about the practical implications of current approaches to the assessment of dangerousness, it should not be read as simply another sociological critique of psychiatric activity. In a larger sense it is a story of all who claim knowledge of human behavior and how some such claims are constructed so as to pass as "expert knowledge," as drawn from resources not possessed by everyone. Thus, it is a story not only of psychiatric experts but of ourselves as well. To miss this point will be to miss what is most essential and most problematic about expertness—that the objectivity of expert knowledge is itself a socially constructed product, and like any other social product has definite moral and political ramifications. This suggestion, while not new, continues to be neglected in most expert work. By raising it now, it is hoped that the reader will carry it as a bookmark in journeying through the following pages, and while examining the production and use of psychiatric realities, dare as well to scrutinize reflexively the construction of other expert knowledge sectors, be they sociological, psychological, biological, economic, or whatever.

I wish to express my gratitude to all of the psychiatric professionals (psychiatrists, psychologists, and social workers) and to the patients who allowed us entry into their work and lives. I genuinely hope that what I have to say about what they have to say will be the basis both for future dialogue and for modest steps toward more humane and just strategies of social control. I also wish to acknowledge my indebtedness to all who collaborated with me in the gathering of data: to Patricia Osher Bresnahan, John Bowman, Susanna Williams, Brunhilde Beitz, Patricia Kochensparger, and Warren Perl. Particular thanks are also given to the readers who have contributed critical and constructive insights to the development of this manuscript: to Gisela Hinkle, Simon Dinitz, and Clyde Franklin for their thorough review of the initial version of this project; to David Orenstein, Ronald Kramer, Judy Golec, Danny Jorgensen, Richard Salem, and Diane Vaughan for their comments and questions throughout; to David Karp, John Johnson, Bob Lavizzo-Mourey, John Conrad, Michele Garvin, and Malcolm Spector for recent suggestions and encouragement.

The research on which this book reports was funded by a grant from the Ohio Division of Mental Health through its Office of Program Evaluation and

Research. I thank that office, and particularly its administrator, Dee Roth, and her assistant, Idona Murray, for their ongoing support and assistance. I finally thank those who have guided this manuscript into its final form: Lorraine Bone, Alice Close, Bertha Shelkan, and Shirley Urban.

# Acknowledgments

Acknowledgment is gratefully made to the following:

Aldine-Atherton Inc., for permission to quote from *Asylums*, by Erving Goffman pp. 155, 159, © 1962 by Aldine Publishing Co., Chicago.

Basic Books, for permission to quote from "The Sociology of Mental Illness," by Alan F. Blum, in *Deviance and Respectability: The Social Construction of Moral Meanings*, edited by Jack D. Douglas, p. 39, © 1970 by Basic Books, Inc., Publishers, New York.

Sage Publications, Inc., for permission to quote from "The 'New Conception of Deviance' and its Critics," by John I. Kituse, in *The Labeling of Deviance: Evaluating a Perspective,* edited by Walter R. Gove, p. 274, © 1976 by Sage Publications, Inc., Beverly Hills, Cal.

Harper and Row Publishers, Inc., for permission to quote from *The Politics of Therapy*, by Seymour L. Halleck, pp. 115, 118, © 1971 by Harper and Row Publishers, New York.

Prentice-Hall, Inc., for permission to quote from *Deviance and Identity*, by John Lofland, p. 136, © 1969, and *Circle of Madness: Being Insane and Institutionalized in America*, by Robert Perrucci, pp. 149-150, © 1974 by Prentice-Hall, Inc., Englewood Cliffs, N.J.

The Society for the Study of Social Problems and the author, for permission to quote from "Negotiating Reality: Notes on Power in the Assessment of Responsibility," by Thomas J. Scheff, 16, 1 (Summer, 1968), pp. 13-14.

Wadsworth Publishing Co., Inc., for permission to quote from *Analyzing Social Settings: Guide to Qualitative Observations and Analysis,* by John Lofland, p. 7, © 1971 by Wadsworth Publishing Co., Inc., Belmont, Cal.

**Part I
Introduction**

# 1

# The Social Construction of Psychiatric Reality: Introducing the Study

*I am not claiming to be a jail house lawyer, all I am trying to do is regain my freedom. My maximum sentence was up five months ago . . . . I don't understand why they insist on fighting my Writ. They have no real grounds to keep me here. All they are doing is prolonging my incarceration unnecessarily.*

From letter of patient-plaintiff in the case of *Davis* v. *Watkins*, April 28, 1972

This book represents a study of the work of a certain kind of social control agent—the "imputational specialist."[1] Although each of us may be concerned with controlling or protecting oneself from the encroachment of those whom he or she perceives deviant, dangerous, or threatening, in modern society it is the imputational specialist who assumes the role of expert classifier, discoverer, diagnoser, or imputer of deviance. One such type of imputational specialist is the psychiatric professional. One of this person's imputational tasks is to assess the mind, emotions, and behaviors of others so as to protect the rest of us from so-called dangerous persons. How exactly such assessments are done and what precisely are the social and political consequences of this type of imputational work are the primary concerns of this book.

Recent developments within both the mental health and criminal justice systems have underscored the need to identify and isolate "dangerous" individuals from others. In the evolution of mental health litigation directed as securing the rights of institutionalized patients the assessment of dangerousness is emerging as the sole criterion by which the state may employ the power of involuntary hospitalization.[2] Within criminal justice circles predictions of dangerousness are being advocated as the primary determinant for the use of imprisonment or as the basis for confining individuals within maximum security facilities. Indeed, the criterion of dangerousness "has been accepted by two national commissions, by the American Law Institute, by the American Bar Association, by the National Council on Crime and Delinquency in its Model Sentencing Act its policy statements, by many commentators and in many criminal codes."[3]

Despite the demand for its employment as a technique of formal social control, the prediction of future dangerousness finds little empirical support. Research on the prediction of violent behavior does not instill confidence in either its reliability or validity. Whether one develops "predictor scales" based on as many as 100 variables[4] or employs the results of psychological testing[5]

3

or relies upon the judgments of experienced diagnosticians,[6] prediction rates rise no higher than two wrong judgments for every one right judgment.[7] A recent review article on this subject has gone so far as to refer to the predictive process as "flipping coins in the courtroom."[8]

In spite of its inadequacies, the assessment of dangerousness is today a mandated responsibility for many psychiatric or mental health professionals. In response to litigative, legislative, and administrative initiatives many psychiatrists, clinical psychologists, and psychiatric social workers are currently engaged in the task of deciding whom it is who tomorrow (or the next day) will be dangerous. How do they make such decisions? In what way, if any, do certain practical, political, and cultural considerations guide their professional work? What concretely constitutes an expert judgment about the "inner psychiatric life" of another so as to declare a person dangerously disturbed? These are important questions which surround the decision to curtail an individual's freedom in order to protect society from the danger that he or she has been diagnosed to represent. In this book these questions are explored through a detailed study of psychiatric decision-makers in action. The present work describes and analyzes what psychiatric professionals actually do when confronted with the task of diagnosing the "psychiatric realities of others" and deciding whom should be confined as dangerous.

## Background to the Study of Court-Ordered
## Assessments of Dangerousness

Lima State Hospital is Ohio's maximum security hospital for the "criminally insane." In the summer of 1974 this institution was the home for approximately 700 extremely marginal individuals. Nearly all came from poor socioeconomic backgrounds. All but about fifty were males. As in other hospitals for the criminally insane, the vast majority of the resident patient-prisoners were white. Blacks have not traditionally made it into hospitals for the criminally insane in the same disproportionate way that they dominate prison populations. Perhaps this reflects some prior judgment by the court system that violent or disruptive blacks are just doing their (subculturally violent) thing, while whites who behave in a similar fashion must be crazy. In any case, the typical Lima patient fit the description of the criminally insane inmate emerging in other research at the time: an extremely marginal white male in his mid-thirties, with few work skills, weak family ties, most likely to have been charged with a crime of violence or (although less likely) charged with some sex offense. In general Lima was popularly believed to house the most dangerous of these persons filtered through the state's criminal justice or mental health systems. It was also the same institution which the *Cleveland Plain Dealer* had several years before branded a "chamber of horrors." Stories about

harsh confinement, brutal beatings, sexual abuse, and the absence of professional treatment had become part of the public record. Convictions had been
sustained against nearly thirty of the hospital's attendant staff for assaults
against patients. It was a "bad" place to be, and a transfer to its maximum
security "medicated" environment was dreaded by inmates in "regular" correctional and mental health institutions.

In September of 1974, a federal district court in Toledo issued an interim
order in major "right-to-treatment" litigation on behalf of all of the hospital's
patients. A major section of this interim order required the state to reevaluate
the status of each patient. These specially contracted psychiatric decision-
makers were grouped into twelve multi-disciplinary review teams. Each review
team consisted of a psychiatrist, a clinical psychologist, and a psychiatric social
worker. Each team was mandated to answer such questions as whether a patient
was mentally ill and/or mentally retarded, dangerous to self or others, and in
need of placement in a maximum security facility. Patients would continue to
be confined in Lima State Hospital only if they were found to be "immediately
dangerous" and needed maximum security or if they were "psychopathic
offenders" requiring further treatment.

The mandate for individual evaluations of the entire Lima State Population
was optimistically received by criminal justice and mental health officials and by
advocates for patients' rights as well. Legal advocates representing the patient-
plaintiffs were confident that the clinicians recruited for these reviews were the
state's "leading experts." According to a Justice Department attorney participating in the case, "The most distinctive part of the order was [that] the Court
required people at Lima to be evaluated against some sort of valid standard for
commitment to see if all patients really belonged there."

The mandate to reevaluate patients also unearthed an enormous clinical
question and a rare opportunity for research. How is it that clinicians actually
do what past research says they should not be able to do (predict dangerousness) and convince themselves and others that they do it well? The Ohio Division
of Mental Health and the clinicians themselves allowed us to study this question.
As the reviews commenced so were we permitted to commence with a field
research project which explored this very issue—the practical production of
diagnostic assessments of dangerousness. Although our specific methods are
presented in greater detail later (Chapter 4), suffice it to say for the present that
a group of seven sociological researchers were able to observe the work of the
twelve teams of psychiatric professionals in 130 diagnostic sessions. After obtaining informed consents, observers situated themselves as unobtrusively as possible in order to note relevant features of social interaction before, during, and
after an evaluation team's interview of patients. In addition to observers' descriptions of this process, tape recordings and transcripts were made of these
selected evaluation sessions.

Furthermore, each participating psychiatric professional was subsequently interviewed regarding his or her impressions, opinions, and reflections concerning both the patient reviews and the presence of the researcher-observers. Together, these materials provide the basis for our analysis of the social dynamics of the psychiatric diagnostic process in the substantive sections of this manuscript.

## Theoretical Focus and Pragmatic Derivatives

A detailed investigation of the process of psychiatric assessment confronts both major theoretical and applied issues. Theoretically, the inquiry represents an examination of certain assumptions associated with the labeling or social reaction perspective on mental illness. This perspective has focused attention on the role of others in categorizing an individual as mentally ill. The recognized existence of deviance, from the labeling perspective, is said to be dependent on the reactions of others. According to Howard Becker, this perspective sensitizes one both to the "larger set of actors" and to "the application of the definition process" by which some behaviors are classified as outside the boundaries of social acceptability.[9] Regarding mental illness, research like that of sociologist Thomas J. Scheff[10] has sought to document the process by which societal reactions organize the "out of touch" behaviors of certain individuals ("residual deviants") into the fixed psychiatric role of the mental patient.

The crucial issue for Scheff and other societal reaction theorists is to outline the social contingencies affecting psychiatric labeling.[11] Controlling efforts for patient behavior have been made to explicate the impact of psychiatric ideology;[12] family preference;[13] the presence of legal advocates;[14] socioeconomic status;[15] and various positive and negative social attributes.[16] Other studies have investigated the relationship between prior labeling and present estimations of illness.[17]

Each study cited above concerns itself with the differential consequences of social variables that lie outside the realm of an individual's behavior. Yet, with several notable exceptions, very little work has been done on the actual interactional procedures by which psychiatrists or other official labelers produce the categorization of mental illness. Scheff provides some illustrative material on interaction in psychiatric interviews[18] and in court psychiatric examination.[19] So do Miller and Schwartz[20] in observations of probate court commitment hearings. More extensive are the descriptions of doctor-patient negotiations of an acceptable diagnosis by Balint,[21] Daniels's account of military psychiatric procedure,[22] Coulter's analysis of the classificatory work of psychiatric social workers,[23] and Perrucci's analysis of mental hospital staffing sessions.[24] Each of these works offers an insight into the actual dynamics of the diagnostic task. The present research seeks to expand these insights through a detailed concern with the process by which psychiatric labels are arrived at and made public. Through extensive field observation, in-depth interviewing, and the analysis of verbatim transcripts it seeks to offer a detailed account of the interactional work that goes into the production of psychiatric diagnosis. Its task is to reconstruct for the reader the procedures by which members of the court-ordered evaluation teams rendered professional interpretations of the psychiatric realities of the patients at Lima State Hospital. Moreover, it focuses on the interactional devices by which evaluators' interpretations are made "objectively" rational and accountable to themselves, to each other, and to the legal agents who commissioned their work.

The concern with the methods that psychiatric team members use to transform private judgments into publicly accountable definitions of deviant reality fosters a direct linkage between labeling or societal reaction theory and that perspective in sociology referred to as ethnomethodology. By ethnomethodology we simply mean the study of the methods that everyday actors employ to convince themselves and to be convincing to others that reality is ordered in a particular fashion, that reality is structured in a particular way. In this study we are concerned then with the methods that psychiatric professionals use to convince themselves and others that the inner (or psychiatric) reality of patients is, in fact, structured in a particular fashion (mentally ill, dangerous, psychopathic, etc.). The usefulness of this linkage between social reaction theory and ethnomethodology will be demonstrated in examining the process by which psychiatric professionals come to recognize other human actors as "mentally ill," as "dangerous," or as "in need of a maximum security environment."

In addition to its theoretical considerations, the present project may be of use to those concerned with the development of mental health policy. The pragmatic advantages here are two-fold. The study first provides mental health officials with concrete data on the diagnostic "criterion-in-use" in actual patient assessments. A comparison of this information with the questions mandated by the court and the answers written up as formal evaluative statements should provide helpful feedback on the manner in which clinicians accomplished their designated mission. Teams fulfilled their mandated objective—the reevaluation of all patients. What about the means they employed in doing the work of patient review? Are these also acceptable to mental health officials and to the legal advocates who brought about the original court action? Specific information on the strategies and criteria employed by the various review teams provides a basis for answering these questions and for anticipating and/or modifying responses to future court actions.

A second applied dimension of this research has as its audience the clinicians who do the work of psychiatric diagnosis. An identification of those social processes that impact on diagnostic procedures and outcomes may provide a reflexive basis for professionals to scrutinize their own behaviors. A clearer understanding of the dynamics of psychiatric interpretation and clinical account-rendering should be helpful to the mental health professional in his or her struggle for maximum objectivity. The advantages here for the mental health system and the adequate treatment of its patients should be obvious.

In summary, in analyzing the actual work of psychiatric imputational specialists we shall explore the theoretical interface between labeling and ethnomethodological perspectives on the sociology of deviance. Moreover, the means used to generate psychiatric evaluations, the impact of social process on clinical decisions, and the negotiated character of predictive indicators are all examined for their applied or pragmatic implications. The following is an outline of the structure by which each of these issues is considered.

## Overview of the Present Work

This report is divided into four parts. Part I is introductory. Part II frames the theoretical and methodological issues involved in doing field research into the process of psychiatric assessment. It comprises three chapters. Chapter 2 examines various sociological considerations of this topic and reviews the literature related to the psychiatric prediction. Factors associated with the invalidity of present predictions are discussed and suggestions are made for a systematic examination of the process of social interaction whence predictions arise. Chapter 3 explicates the conceptual framework by which the study approaches the social generation of psychiatric decisions. The usefulness of the ethnomethodological approach to this topic is assessed and a theoretical framework for analyzing the diagnostic work of psychiatric team members is presented. In Chapter 4 the methods of data-gathering and analysis are described. Particular attention is paid to the role of the field researcher in observing and rendering accounts of social interaction.

Part II represents the substantive consideration of the work of patient review. It involves five chapters. The first (Chapter 5) presents some background on the major actors involved in the diagnostic process: the psychiatric professionals and their patients. It additionally discusses the manner in which review team members were recruited and prepared for their diagnostic task. The analysis of the interactional work involved in reviewing patients is the focus of Chapters 6 through 9. Chapter 6 provides a somewhat holistic view of the process of patient review. It examines the "purposes-at-hand" that guided team member interaction and the manner in which teams thematized operating definitions of such things as mental illness, dangerousness, and psychopathy. Chapter 7 describes and analyzes the "previewing of patients" prior to the psychiatric interview. The manner in which teams orient themselves to their own mission and ways in which they establish a sense of "typical" records and "types" of actors are focal concerns of this chapter. Chapter 8, on the other hand, focuses on the conversational features of diagnostic interviews and on the processes by which teams "discover" and "document" psychiatric evidence. The postviewing of patients in discussion subsequent to the diagnostic interview is the topic of Chapter 9. The procedures by which teams came to and objectify their decisions is the subject for analysis in this chapter.

The analysis of the properties and process of psychiatric diagnosis is accompanied by detailed description of and direct quotations from the interactions of the patient review teams. Its objective is to realize a sociological understanding of the work by which diagnostic actors construct accounts of the psychiatric realities of others. The theoretical and applied implications of viewing diagnostic work as a practical social accomplishment are discussed in Part IV. The overriding issue here, as in the work as a whole, concerns the process by which it is determined that an individual is mentally disordered, dangerous, and needs or does not need the confines of a maximum security mental hospital. The political and moral dimensions of this question should be evident. What is really being examined, after all, is the process by which it is professionally decided to curtail one individual's present freedom for the purpose of safeguarding another individual's future safety.

## Notes

1. The term "imputational specialist," implying a professional commitment to ensuring a regular flow of social deviance, is borrowed from John Lofland, *Deviance and Identity* (Englewood Cliffs, N.J.: Prentice-Hall, 1969), p. 139.

2. For a more general discussion of the emerging importance of "dangerousness" as the sole criterion for involuntary commitment see Stephen J. Pfohl, *Right to Treatment Litigation: A Consideration of Judicial Intervention into Mental Health Policy* (Columbus, Ohio: Ohio Division of Mental Health, 1975); and Alan A. Stone, *Mental Health and Law: A System in Transition* (Rockville, Md.: National Institute of Mental Health, 1975).

3. Norval Morris. *The Future of Imprisonment* (Chicago: University of Chicago Press, 1974), pp. 62-63.

4. E. Wenk, J. Robison, and G. Smith, "Can Violence Be Predicted?" *Crime and Delinquency* 18 (1972): 393-402.

5. E. Megargee, "The Prediction of Violence with Psychological Tests," in C. Speilberger, ed., *Current Topics in Clinical and Community Psychology* (New York: The Academic Press, 1970), pp. 98-156.

6. H.R. Kozol, R. Boucher, and R. Garofalo, "The Diagnosis and Treatment of Dangerousness," *Crime and Delinquency* 18 (1972): 371-392; H. Steadman and J. Cocozza, *Careers of the Criminally Insane: Excess Social Control of Deviance* (Lexington, Mass.: Lexington Books, 1974).

7. Actually rates are usually considerably lower. The "maximum rate"

referred to here would entail the retention of all "criminally insane" or "foren-sic" patients under age fifty, while still incurring a 2-1 ratio of false positive predictions (see Steadman and Cocozza, 1974). Other studies have found the false prediction rate to be as high as 95 percent (Wenk, Robison, and Smith, 1972).

8. Bruce J. Ennis and Thomas R. Litwack, "Psychiatry and the Presumption of Expertise: Flipping Coins in the Courtroom," *California Law Review* 62 (May 1974): 693-752.

9. Howard S. Becker, "Labelling Theory Reconsidered," in H. Becker, *Outsiders: Studies in the Sociology of Deviance* (New York: The Free Press, 1973), pp. 177-208.

10. Thomas J. Scheff, *Being Mentally Ill: A Sociological Theory* (Chicago: Aldine, 1966).

11. Thomas J. Scheff, "The Labelling Theory of Mental Illness", *American Sociological Review* 3a (June 1974): 444-452.

12. Thomas J. Scheff, "The Societal Reaction to Deviance: Ascriptive Elements in the Psychiatric Screening of Mental Patients in a Midwestern State," *Social Problems* 11 (Spring 1964): 401-413.

13. James R. Greenley, "The Psychiatric Patient's Family and the Length of Hospitalization," *Journal of Health and Social Behavior* 13 (March 1972): 25-37.

14. Dennis R. Wegner and C. Richard Fletcher, "The Effect of Legal Counsel on Admissions to a State Mental Hospital: A Confrontation of Professions," *Journal of Health and Social Behavior* 10 (June 1969): 349-353.

15. Arnold S. Linsky, "Community Homogeneity and Exclusion of the Mentally Ill: Rejection v. Consensus About Deviance," *Journal of Health and Social Behavior* 14 (December 1970): 304-311. William A. Rushing, "Legitimate, Transitional and Illegitimate Mental Patients in a Midwestern State," *American Journal of Sociology* 77 (November 1971): 511-526.

16. William A. Wilde, "Decision-Making in a Psychiatric Screening Agency," *Journal of Health and Social Behavior* 9 (September 1968): 215-221. Arnold S. Linsky, "Who Shall Be Excluded: The Influence of Personal Attributes in Community Reactions to the Mentally Ill," *Social Psychiatry* 5 (July 1970): 166-171.

17. Maurice K. Temerlin, "Suggestion Effects in Psychiatric Diagnosis," *Journal of Nervous and Mental Disease* 147 (April 1968): 349-353. David L. Rosenhan, "On Being Sane in Insane Places," *Science* 179 (January 1973): 250-258.

18. Thomas J. Scheff, "Negotiating Reality on Power in the Assessment of Responsibility," *Social Problems* 16 (Summer 1968): 3-17.

19. Thomas J. Scheff, *Being Mentally Ill.*

20. Dorothy Miller and Michael Schwartz, "County Lunacy Commission

Hearings: Some Observations of Commitments to a State Mental Hospital," *Social Problems* 14 (Summer 1966): 26-35.

21. Michael Balint, *The Doctor, His Patient and the Illness* (New York: International Universities Press, 1957).

22. Arlene Daniels, "The Social Construction of Psychiatric Diagnosis," in H. Dreitzel, *Recent Sociology No. 2* (New York: Macmillan, 1970), pp. 182-205.

23. Jeff Coulter, *The Operations of Mental Health Personnel in an Urban Area* (Manchester, England: University of Manchester, unpublished dissertation, 1975).

24. Robert Perrucci, *Circle of Madness: Being Insane and Institutionalized in America* (Englewood Cliffs, N.J.: Prentice-Hall, 1974).

**Part II
Theory and Methods**

# 2

## Framing the Study: Theoretical Considerations

*There is, of course, considerable value to diagnosis in ordinary medical practice. Putting people into diagnostic categories makes it convenient for doctors to communicate with one another and enables research to be done. . . . In psychiatry, however, diagnostic categories such as schizophrenia, paranoia, psychopathy, or alcoholism are not sufficiently precise so that the doctor can have a clear idea of desirable treatment or prognosis. . . . Psychiatrists could help society immeasurably. . . if they would frankly admit that current diagnostic categories do not have much scientific meaning—that they are largely arbitrary. Then society might be able to confront rationally and humanely the moral questions raised by those who behave differently.*

Seymour L. Halleck, *The Politics of Therapy* (New York: Harper and Row, 1971), pp. 115, 118

How reliable are psychiatric assessments of mental disorders, dangerousness, and the need for hospitalized confinement? To what degree will such assessments be consistent between diagnosers or between an initial and subsequent diagnosis? How valid are these judgments? To what degree do they classify and predict that which they claim to classify and predict? Given the significance of psychiatric decision-making as a form of social control, these are important questions. They are also questions which have been the subject of a considerable body of research. This chapter briefly surveys the basic findings of this research and reviews a set of sociological interpretations regarding the inadequacy of psychiatric decision-making. The dominant assumptions guiding past research are then compared with the theoretical concerns of the present investigation. A contrast is made between what will be referred to as the postulate of "subjective distortion" in most past work and the postulate of "mutual determination" in our own. The chapter concludes with the introduction of our conceptual framework for studying the actual work of psychiatric assessments.

### Questioning the Adequacy of Psychiatric Decision-Making

Past studies of psychiatric decision-making provide little confidence in the reliability or validity of diagnosing mental illness and predicting its consequences (that is, dangerousness, need for confinement, etc.). Actually, the entire system of diagnostic classification (sorting persons into various disease types and sub-types) has come under attack during recent years from several perspectives. The political and ethical underside of psychiatric categorization has been scored by psychiatrist Szasz. In debunking the "myth of mental illness," Szasz argues that to classify psychiatric disorders as disease entities is to distort the social fact that "the finding of mental illness is made by establishing a deviance in behavior from certain psychosocial, ethical, or legal norms."[1] Sociologists such as Scheff have also criticized the system for bypassing the social process whereby individuals, who break everyday norms governing recognized standards of decency and appropriate displays of reality, are labeled as mentally ill.[2] The existential problems arising from the application of diseaselike nomenclature has similarly been criticized by R.D. Laing and his associates. They maintain that diagnostic categorization falsifies the willful and intentional quality of much creative human experience.[3] From quite another perspective, psychiatric classifications are criticized by behaviorists who view "maladaptive" behaviors as learned patterns of human response rather than as symptoms of some illness or disease of the mind.[4]

Despite the global objections to current diagnostic practice, research has pointed to the resurgence of traditional diagnostic categories in recent years.[5] Other work suggests that this renewed confidence in traditional psychiatric nomenclature has been generated by a variety of biological and genetic studies (particularly those of psychoses), and by belief in the medical effectiveness of psychotropic drugs.[6] While these developments may support a general faith in the illness conception of mental disorders, they do little actually to refine the diagnostic techniques of clinicians in day-to-day practice. That is to say that the biologic-genetic determination of "mental disease" resides largely in the world of research, while the postdiagnostic control of "symptoms" with psychotherapeutic drugs has little to do with the recognition and categorization of symptomatic behavior in the first place. Studies of actual diagnostic practice, however, consistently document the unreliability of clinical judgments and the invalidity of psychiatric classification. While it is beyond the scope of the present work to provide a detailed (study by study) examination of this previous research, in the following paragraphs we shall outline the major conclusions suggested by these investigations.

*The Unreliability of Psychiatric Diagnoses*

Joseph Zubin, in a detailed review of literature in this area, concludes that, while clinicians show some agreement with regard to general categories of diagnosis (that is, agreement ranging from 64-84 percent), "the degree of over-all agreement between different observers with regard to specific diagnoses is too low for individual diagnosis."[7] Moreover, Zubin argues that the low levels of agreement for specific diagnosis are all the more surprising, given that raters in these studies were ordinarily extremely similar in professional orientation, background, and training. Other reviews reached very similar conclusions. Ennis and Litwack state simply "that psychiatric diagnoses using these [traditional diagnostic] categories are not very reliable."[8] According to Ziskin, the most typical research results suggest that, on the average, one cannot expect to find agreement between two psychiatrists in more than about 60 percent of cases.[9] Ziskin states that the probability that a second clinician will agree with the diagnosis of a first is "barely better than 50-50," and that "there is about as much chance that a different expert would come to some different conclusion as there is that the other would agree."[10] When one excludes diagnoses of organic impairments, upon which there is more agreement, the reliability of psychiatric decisions is said to drop to around 40 percent.[11]

*The Validity of Diagnoses*

The problems encountered regarding the reliability of psychiatric diagnoses are multiplied when one considers the validity of these procedures. By validity is meant the degree to which diagnoses measure what they purport to measure. The most immediate problem here is definitional. That which is ideally to be measured is hardly an agreed-upon phenomenon. As alluded to previously, the whole problem of mental illness has been redefined by critics of the so-called medical model. Rather than conceiving of mental disorders as a catalogue of diseases, critics have suggested a reformulation in terms of "problems with living,"[12] arising in a "distorted nexus of human communication,"[13] resulting in the labeling of "residual deviants"[14] and in their subsequent "victimization" by agents of social control.[15]

Even for those who adhere to the assumptions of the illness model, the definitional problem is far from resolved. What is lacking in the system of psychiatric classification is a clear set of operational definitions or indicators by which the various subtypes of a disease entity may be recognized and unambiguously diagnosed. Without such conceptual and operational clarity the issue of validity will never be resolved.[16] Moreover, without this clarity it is not surprising that rates of diagnostic reliability are so consistently low.

Even of the lack of operational clarity in psychiatric diagnosis is provided by Zubin in his discussion of "the absence of relationships between diagnoses and symptomatology" (the operational definitions of mental illness).[17] Zubin discusses the results of a study by Freudenberg and Robertson[18] which found considerable overlap of symptoms among the various diagnostic categories. Such a finding is said to undermine the "concurrent validity" of diagnoses (the substantiation of diagnostic categories by measures independent of the categories themselves). If the "independent measures" are not exclusive between categories, upon what basis are psychiatric decisions made? This question is compounded by the work of Zigler and Philips, which also uncovered low relationships between symptoms and diagnoses.[19] Likewise, Katz and his associates conclude that diagnostic categories are not specific for configurations or "patterns of symptomatology,"[20] Yet, suggests Zubin, aside from the search for symptoms in clinical interviewing, the practicing diagnostician has little else to aid him in his work. Zubin's review of psychometric inventories (such as the MMPI) and projective tests suggests that these measures offer little in terms of uncontaminated concurrent corroboration of diagnoses.[21] On the other hand, the independent substantiation "of diagnoses emanating from biochemical, physiological, sensory, perceptual, and psychomotor techniques [is] still so embryonic" that it is said to have little impact on the day-to-day practice of psychiatric decision-making.[22]

In summary, definitional uncertainties and operational inadequacies undermine the validity of current diagnostic practice. Yet, the simple recognition of mental disorders is not the only purpose of psychiatric diagnosis. Psychiatric decisions are also relied upon to predict future dangerousness and hence determine a patient's need for future hospitalization. This predictive task was, of course, the major responsibility assigned to the psychiatric evaluation teams at Lima State Hospital. How valid is the process of diagnosis in measuring this phenomenon?

*The Validity of Psychiatric Predictions of Dangerousness*

The clinical prediction of dangerousness is also of questionable validity. Most research shows that psychiatric professionals, in fact, have little ability to predict validly who will act in violent or dangerous manner. As inaccurate as predictions may be, equally problematic is the direction in which they consistently err—error through over-prediction. Indeed, in study after study, the same conclusion emerges: that for every one correct psychiatric prediction of violence, there are numerous incorrect predictions. Thus, according to Dershowitz, among all of those presently confined on the basis of psychiatric predictions of violence, "there are a few who would, and many more who would not, actually engage in such conduct if released."[23]

Conclusions regarding inaccuracy and overprediction in the diagnosis are grounded in a number of empirical investigations. Wenk, Robison, and Smith report on three such research efforts.[24] They first attempted to develop a "violence predictor scale" which would aid parole decision-making. Using such "predictive items" as commitment offense, number of prior commitments, opiate use, and length of imprisonment the researchers identified a small class of offenders who could be expected to be violent. However, of those identified as potentially violent, 85 percent never committed a violent act while on parole.

In a second study, offender histories and psychiatric reports were used to assign 7,712 parolees to categories reflecting their potentiality for violence. The use of these indicators was even more alarming. For each correct identification of a potentially aggressive individual there were 326 incorrect identifications. The third study utilized 100 possibly predictive variables, including extensive social-historical background information results of psychiatric diagnoses and the findings of psychological testing, in a fifteen-month follow-up of 4,146 wards of the California Youth Authority. The best simple indicator of future violence was the use of a history of actual violence as a sole predictor. Yet even this measure resulted in nineteen false positives for every twenty predictions. Different multivariate regression equations were also employed in analyzing the impact of the 100 variables. The best of these, however, could do no better than to produce eight false predictions for every one accurate prediction.

A five-year follow-up of patients released from the Massachusetts Center for the Diagnosis and Treatment of Dangerous Persons by Kozol, Boucher, and Garofalo revealed a slightly better rate of predictive accuracy.[25] Recommendations were made for retention or release on the basis of independent examinations of each patient by at least two psychiatrists, two psychologists, and one social worker. Furthermore, each examination included a full battery of psychological tests, and a rigorous attempt to reconstruct a person's life history, based on data from the patient, family, friends, neighbors, teachers, employers and court, correctional and mental hospital records.

Of 435 releases during a ten-year period, forty-nine were made against the recommendations of Kozol and his associates. Of these (predicted as dangerous yet released), 34.7 percent committed serious assaultive acts during the five-year follow-up period. When this figure is compared to the 8 percent of the releases who were assessed as nondangerous and committed similar acts of violence, the assessment of dangerousness appears to have some validity. It should be remembered, however, that 65 percent of the individuals labeled as dangerous did not later commit a violent act. Hence, in spite of the extensive use of multiple examiners, data sources, and testing, two out of every three predictions of violence were wrong. Similar findings were evidenced in a follow-up of residents at Maryland's Patuxent Institution, where a comparison of staff recommendations with later recidivism yielded false positives at the rate of 54 percent.[26] Moreover, Megargee's extensive review of the use of psychological testing in the prediction of violent behavior led to the conclusion that no instrument has been developed which adequately *postdicts,* let alone *predicts*, violent behavior.[27]

Perhaps the most telling evidence about the inadequacy of predictive practice comes from a four-year follow-up of *Baxstrom* patients by Steadman and Cocozza.[28] These patients were transferred from two New York State "hospitals for the criminally insane" as a result of the previously discussed *Baxstrom* decision. Since all patients had been previously retained because they were presumed to be dangerous and in need of maximum security, their release provided a rare opportunity for naturalistic research on the validity of predictions of dangerousness. The results of this study confirm what we have already noted about this issue—inaccuracy and overprediction. During the four-year follow-up only 20 percent of this supposedly dangerous population were ever assaultive of another individual in either a civilian hospital or in the community. Of those 927 transferred to lesser restrictive hospitals only twenty-seven were returned to the maximum security hospital for the criminally insane. Of those eventually released to the community only 20 percent were rearrested. Practically all of these arrests were for "nuisance crimes" like vagrancy and intoxication. Only 5 percent were arrested for felonies. In addition, the two factors most closely associated with recidivism or rehospitalization, age and severity of criminal history, still resulted in two false predictions for every one correct prediction. Moreover, this problematic rate of prediction could only be achieved by constructing the age variable so as to include all patients fifty years or younger in the same category. Thus, to act on this predictive information would mean to retain custody of all patients under age fifty (most patients), while still incurring a 2-1 ratio of false positive predictions.

Each of the research efforts described above support the contention that predictions of dangerousness have been consistently characterized by low levels of validity. This finding is even more striking considering the fact that the populations for the various studies were systematically biased in the direction of positive results. The various research subjects were, after all, primarily convicted offenders, "sexual psychopaths," and adjudicated delinquents. Yet, even for this highly eschewed sample the rates of false positives ran between 54 and 99 percent. This problematic conclusion is summarized by Monahan, who suggests that violence is vastly overpredicted, regardless of whether one relies on psychological testing and in-depth psychiatric examinations, on simple behavioral indicators, or on sophisticated multivariate research design.[29]

**Sociological Accounts of the Inadequacy of Psychiatric Decision-Making**

Much sociological reasoning has been directed toward explanatory accounts of the unreliability and invalidity of psychiatric decision-making. According to Coulter, "Most, if not all, of the studies of diagnostic activities in psychiatry conducted by sociologists in recent years have sought to theorize about the organizational and ideological 'contaminations' considered to play decisive parts in the actual formulations of psychiatric diagnoses."[30] The well-known work of Scheff is a clear example of this type of sociological accounting. His investigations suggest that such organizational factors as the brevity of interview time, the vagueness of legal criteria, the inadequacies of patient records, beliefs concerning limited quotas for release of patients, and financial rewards for rapid processing all contribute to "the gross unreliability of psychiatric diagnosis as an indication of anything about the behavior of the patient."[31] On the other hand, low levels of validity are conceived as related to the social and economic marginality of patients, the relative independence that diagnosticians have in relation to their clients, insubstantive knowledge concerning the believed etiology of mental diseases, and the socialization of clinicians into stereotypical rules for proficiently recognizing "normal cases."[32]

Scheff's findings also describe the impact of various social contingencies independent of the assessed seriousness of a patient's mental disorder or of his or her dangerousness. Controlling for the latter variables, a patient's age and length of confinement, and the type of hospital in which he or she was institutionalized were seen to be significant determinants of the likelihood for or against release.[33] The distortion of diagnostic information by family members seeking a patient's institutionalization has also been discussed. Families (and those considered to be significant others) are said frequently to present hostile or confused accounts which conflict with patients' descriptions of their own behavior. Hence one often observes three separate versions of so-called psychiatric symptoms: that of the family, that of the patient, and that of the diagnostician.[34]

The routine "assumption of illness" and belief in the "medical model" are also said to produce overly conservative patterns of psychiatric judgments. While researchers like Mechanic attribute these biasing elements to the professional socialization of psychiatrists as physicians and to the time-limited demands of the institutional work structure,[35] Scheff extends his analysis to identify financial, ideological, and political sources of distortion.[36] Financially diagnosers are said to have incentives to process cases overly quickly since they are ordinarily paid on a per-case basis. Ideologically, several cognitive features of the so-called medical model are said to buttress the assumption that a patient is "in fact" ill. One of the most important of these suggests that, like other disease entities, mental illness, if undetected and untreated, will increase in seriousness and result in further mental deterioration. A second assumes that diagnosis is not an irreversible act, and that, relative to the dangers resulting from the disease, psychiatric classification and treatment are either helpful or neutral. Like these ideological contaminations, certain political pressures were also described as promoting a "better safe than sorry" policy of conservative judgments. These pressures concerned diagnosticians' beliefs as to the severity of sanctions for erroneously releasing persons who would later act dangerously, when contrasted to the weakness of any sanctions for erroneously retaining the nondangerous.

A number of other sociological formulations of the inadequacy of diagnostic procedures supplement the organizational, financial, ideological, and political biases discussed by Scheff. Ennis and Litwack group these biases into six categories and review numerous studies which contribute to the recognition of each.[37] For our purposes it will suffice to list these categorical headings and the kinds of contaminants subsumed by each. They include biases stemming from (1) clinical orientation and training (that is, professional socialization into often competing or contradictory clinical belief systems); (2) the context of psychiatric decision-making (that is, the impact of prior information, political and organizational pressures, and the removal of individuals from the usual "scenes" of their psychiatric troubles; (3) the timing of diagnosis (that is, problems with one-time samplings); (4) class and cultural variables (for example, distortion by virtue of economic, radical, gender, or cultural stereotyping); (5) personal clinical preferences (that is, factors related to idiosyncratic biases of a diagnoser's orientation, personality, defensiveness, etc.); (6) inadequacies in the formal diagnostic system (definitional ambiguity, the problem of inferring states of being from single symptoms, etc.).

In addition to the contamination factors suggested above, Monahan suggests that the lack of corrective feedback (on diagnostician inaccuracy), differential consequences to the subject (that is, the desire to obtain a certain treatment modality for a particular patient), the problem of "illusory correlation" (that is, systematically "seeing" relationships between classes of events where no such relationships actually exist), the existence of low base-rates of violence (that is, the problem of predicting rarely occurring events), and the powerlessness of subjects to resist diagnostic labeling are all further factors which cloud the accurate assessment of dangerousness in particular.[38]

### Psychiatric Decision-Making: The Interactional Work

The previous discussion has reviewed numerous criticisms of the reliability and validity of psychiatric decision-making. These have ranged from global philosophical objections to inferences drawn from detailed empirical studies suggesting social and psychological obstacles to the objectivity of psychiatric judgments. If psychiatric diagnosis is "underdeveloped" in the present, what would it look like if it were fully "developed"? An answer to this question is found in a further consideration of the critical research described above. A more idealized state of diagnosis would seemingly be a more rationalized state.[39] It would be a state in which the ends of the diagnostic process (a recognition of a particular disease entity and its consequences) would be reliably and validly ascertained by *means* of an objective and unbiased system of decision-making rules. If these rules were properly followed, the objectives of diagnosis would be realized. This idealized state of affairs implies an idealization of the notion of rationality. The decision-maker in this model would be much like the computer which, when it follows the prescribed program, produces the desired information.

The "idealized" state of affairs is not realized in the "real" world of psychiatric decision-making. This is the conclusion of the body of research surveyed above. This research presents a picture of "nonrationality" rather than "idealized rationality." The whole process of psychiatric decision-making is portrayed as tainted, biased, or distorted by such social factors as "context," "training," "timing," and "cultural differences," and by such psychological factors as "the differential consequences to diagnostician or subject" and the "problem of illusory correlation." These factors plague the process of diagnosis and are compounded by such things as a lack of clear etiological knowledge and definitional preciseness. All of these variables combine to give psychiatric decision-making the appearance of "ad hoc" nonrationality rather than characteristics of objective rationality. The ends of diagnosis cannot be efficiently and effectively achieved because too many factors are said to disturb and distort the means.

Although most studies of psychiatric decision-making seek to document its nonrationality, they do not appear to abandon the premise that it should, in principle, be characterized by an idealized rationality. In this sense the studies take on the character of being exposés or critiques of the objectivity of psychiatric judgments.[40] Besides exposing the social and psychological nonrationality of the diagnostic process, the studies (at least implicitly) offer mechanisms of reform. Such mechanisms are believed to reduce bias and distortion so that psychiatric judgments may better approximate the characteristic of idealized rationality. Hence, factors such as bias by training, timing, or context appear to be delineated in order that they may be overcome and psychiatric judgments may be more objective. To eliminate much of the taint of subjectivity researchers have proposed standardizing all diagnostic procedures[41] or even developing computerized diagnostic packages.[42] Such mechanisms would restore the rational means-end character of diagnosis by reducing the "ad hoc" nature of its present social and psychological biases.

The "exposé-reformist" style of research has been helpful in delineating variables which may account for the apparent arbitrariness of much psychiatric decision-making. An outline of these variables may sensitize clinicians to factors which influence their perceptions and evaluations of patients. From another perspective, however, this research may be said to be considerably lacking. It provides a critical comparison between the idealized rational nature of diagnosis and the actual state of affairs in the field today. It does not provide an account of how "contaminating factors" actually emerge as elements in the concrete interactional work of clinicians themselves. In what ways, if any, do those things which appear as irrational distortions to the researcher become rational (that is, acceptable, accountable, logical, and noncontradictory) for diagnosers? This question reminds one of Garfinkel's observation that most social scientists "have preferred . . . to study the features and conditions of nonrationality in human conduct," rather than to investigate the social procedures that actors use to accomplish a sense of rational order in everyday life.[43]

A focus on the social procedures that clinicians use to accomplish psychiatric diagnoses is missing in most of the research described to this point. In other words, most research has paid little attention to the interaction whereby psychiatric judgments emerge as concrete products of social actors. We are told by past research that one's clinical training influences what one is likely to see in a patient's behavior. We are not informed about how the categories of a particular clinical orientation are situationally employed to make sense of what a patient is doing or saying. We are told that knowledge of past diagnoses may bias present judgments. We are not informed about how past "types" of any sort of knowledge are paired with perceptions of patients in a particular context to accomplish attributions of mental illness. We are told that differential consequences for the subject may distort the accuracy in the prediction of dangerousness. We are not informed about how "typical" knowledge of differential consequences specifically functions to remove the contradictions involved in classifying an individual according to a category to which he or she "really doesn't belong." Moreover, we are told very little about the contextbound process of interaction whereby professionals produce diagnostic categorizations which they recognize as rational, as accurate, and to which patients "really do belong." Hence, in the words of Coulter, these past research efforts do little "to preserve for their readers any empirical features of the interactional episodes or sequences constituting 'diagnostic work' as a course of action."[44]

Knowing about the specific social interactions that lead to a psychiatric decision is essential in order to have the clearest understanding of what diagnostic judgments are actually all about. Is the idealized rationality of the medical model the most useful vehicle for understanding what psychiatric diagnosis is in practice? Are such things as the impact of past records, context, timing, and training really distortions of an otherwise rational relationship between means and ends, between "ways of looking" and the results of seeing what is "really there"? Or is the "reality" of what is there (the recognized existence of a mental disease) better understood as the product of looking in particular ways? In other words, are the diagnostic uses of such things as past records, context, timing, and training intrinsic to, rather than distortive of, the process of psychiatric decision-making?

If the answer to the preceding question is affirmative, we must employ a different set of strategies for improving the process of psychiatric decision-making. It becomes useless to talk of ways of getting around the contextbound limitations of diagnosis. The context and all the social and psychological factors, previously discussed as being distortive, become constitutive elements in the process whereby some actors (diagnosticians) size up and apply diagnostic labels to other actors (patients). The improvement of diagnosis would thus imply constructive attempts to use or control the impact of contextual variables rather than to eliminate them. The question as to which model represents a better understanding of the concreteness of psychiatric diagnosis cannot, however, be answered by a review of the past research. This research, afterall, operates on the assumption that the social processes compromise rather than constitute the objectivity of psychiatric decision-making. What is needed is detailed study of the actual role of social interaction in generating psychiatric judgments. Only then can we hope to determine whether the social process is extrinsic and distortive or intrinsic and essential to the categorical evaluation of another's psychiatric reality.

In contrast to most past efforts, the present study of psychiatric assessment study does not assume that the "ad hoc" features of psychiatric diagnosis are factors which bias the idealized rationality of the decision-making process. It inquires, instead, into the question of whether "ad hoc" procedures constitute the essential core of the process of diagnosis. Rather than representing yet another critique of the failure of diagnostic work to achieve idealized rationality, this research is designed as a study of the success of the work of diagnosis in achieving what Schutz referred to as "everyday" or "practical rationality." As distinct from a means-end, computerlike model of rationality, everyday rationality connotes the process by which actors utilize typified stocks of knowledge and recipes for social action, within the constraints of particular contexts, in order to produce the appearance (both for themselves and others) that their decisions are "reasonable," "proper," "logical," "acceptable," "legal," and so forth.[45] In the case of psychiatric decision-making, we are interested in the interactional process whereby clinicians produce apparently acceptable professional categorizations of a patient's mental state, and in the process used to accomplish their own accepted identities as professional diagnosticians.

Another way of framing the interests of the present study is to return to the distinction between diagnostic procedures as represented by various "ways of looking," and diagnostic findings as indicative of the results of seeing what is "really there." Past research has typically inferred the inadequacy of the procedures by assessing the objectivity of the findings. When various clinicians see what is "really there" in an inconsistent manner or when their seeing demonstrates little relationship to a patient's future behavior, it is concluded that the "ways of looking" must have been distorted or biased. This interpretation assumes that there is something "really there," to be seen independent of the "ways of looking." An alternative interpretation is that the procedures and findings, the "ways of looking" and the "results of seeing," are mutually determinative. This is to say that there can be nothing "really there" except for that which is the product of the "ways of looking" and that there can be no "ways of looking" except for those that are guided by the manner in which something is "really there" in an actor's stock of typified knowledge. Hence, this alternative interpretation assumes no independence of procedures and findings.

The first of the two interpretations described above will be referred to as the "subjective distortion" interpretation. This interpretation reasons that numerous dimensions of a diagnostician's subjectivity and of the decision-making context distort or bias the objectivity of a psychiatric diagnosis. The second interpretation will be referred to as the "mutually determinative" interpretation. It reasons that a diagnostician's subjectivity and context interact with typified knowledge about a particular patient to produce the appearance of objectivity for a psychiatric diagnosis.

The first interpretation is supported by the numerous reliability and validity studies discussed in this chapter. These studies have concentrated on analyzing the adequacy of the results of seeing what is "really there." They have paid little attention to the concrete procedures involved in the "ways of (diagnostic) looking." These studies have focused on what Kaplan calls the "reconstructed logic" (of psychiatric decision-making), while neglecting the "logic-in-use" (in the process of diagnosis itself).[46] On the other hand, an adequate exploration of the "mutually determinative" interpretation requires a detailed examination of the interrelationships between these two types of logic, between the "ways of knowing" and the "results of seeing." Such an examination is the goal of the present study. It concentrates specifically on the interactional work involved in psychiatric diagnosis, on the social procedures by which a diagnostician's subjectivity and context are concretely related to the "objectivity" of diagnostic findings. In so doing, the study contrasts and compares the "subjective distortion interpretation" with the "mutually determinative interpretation" of psychiatric decision-making.

## Notes

1. Thomas Szasz, "The Myth of Mental Illness," in S. Spitzer and N. Denzin, eds., *The Mental Patient: Studies in the Sociology of Deviance* (New York: McGraw-Hill Book Co., 1968), p. 25.

2. Thomas J. Scheff, "The Role of the Mentally Ill and the Dynamics of Mental Disorder: A Research Framework," in S. Spitzer and N. Denzin, eds. *The Mental Patient: Studies in the Sociology of Deviance* (New York: McGraw-Hill Book Co., 1968), pp. 8-22.

3. R.D. Laing and A. Esterson, *Sanity, Madness and the Family* (Baltimore, Md.: Penguin Books, 1964); R.D. Laing, *The Politics of Experience* (New York: Ballantine Books, 1967).

4. Leonard P. Ullmann and Leonard Krasner, *A Psychological Approach to Abnormal Behavior* (Englewood Cliffs; N.J.: Prentice-Hall, 1969); Albert Bandura, *Principles of Behavior Modification* (New York: Holt, Rinehart, and Winston, 1969; Ronald L. Akers, *Deviant Behavior: A Social Learning Approach* (Belmont, Cal.: Wadsworth Publishing Co., Inc., 1973).

5. Leslie Phillips and Juris G. Draguns, "Classification of the Behavioral Disorders," *Annual Review of Psychology* 22 (1971): 447-482.

6. Alan A. Stone, *Mental Health and Law: A System in Transition* (Rockville, Md.: National Institute of Mental Health, 1975), p. 65.

7. Joseph Zubin, "Classification of the Behavioral Disorders," *Annual Review of Psychology* 18 (1967): 383. Zubin's comprehensive review of this subject considers both "agreement" reliability (agreement in classification between two or more observers) and "consistency" reliability (agreement between an initial and subsequent diagnosis). His analysis and that of the other reviews cited in this section cover such major studies as P. Ash, "The Reliability of Psychiatric Diagnosis," *Journal of Abnormal and Social Psychology* 44 (1949): 272-76; H.O. Schmidt and C.P. Fonda, "The Reliability of Psychiatric Diagnosis: A New Look," *Journal of Abnormal and Social Psychology* 52 (1956): 262-267; V. Norris, *Mental Illness in London Maudsley Monographs No. 6* (London: Chapman & Hall, 1959), pp. 42-53; A.T. Beck et al., "Reliability of Psychiatric Diagnosis: A Study of Consistency of Clinical Judgments and Ratings," *American Journal of Psychiatry* 119A (October 1962): 351-557; B. Mehlman, "The Reliability of Psychiatric Diagnoses," *Journal of Abnormal and Social Psychology* 47 (1952): 577; Benjamin Pasamanick, Simon Dinitz, and Mark Lefton, "Psychiatric Orientation and Its Relation to Diagnosis and Treatment in a Mental Hospital," *American Journal of Psychiatry* 116 (1959): 127-132; Martin M. Katz, Jonathan O. Cole, and Henri A. Lowery, "Studies of the Diagnostic Process: The Influence of Symptom Perception, Past Experience, and Ethnic Background in Diagnostic Decisions," *American Journal of Psychiatry* 125, 7 (February 1969): 937-947.

8. Bruce J. Ennis and Thomas R. Litwack, "Psychiatry and the Presumption of Expertise: Flipping Coins in the Courtroom," *California Law Review* 62, 3 (May 1974): 701.

9. Jay Ziskin, *Coping with Psychiatric and Psychological Testimony* (Beverly Hills, Cal.: Law and Psychology Press, 1970), p. 123.

10. Ibid., p. 126.

11. Ennis and Litwack, p. 702.

12. Thomas Szasz, "The Myth of Mental Illness," *The American Psychologist* 15 (February 1960): 113-118.

13. R.D. Laing and A. Esterson, *Sanity, Madness and the Family.*

14. Thomas J. Scheff, *Being Mentally Ill: A Sociological Theory* (Chicago: Aldine, 1966).

15. Robert Perrucci, *Circle of Madness: Being Insane and Institutionalized in America* (Englewood Cliffs, N.J.: Prentice-Hall, 1974).

16. The importance of independent operational definitions of the phenomenon to be measured is outlined in A. Kaplan's *The Conduct of Inquiry: Methodology for Behavioral Sciences* (Scranton, Pa.: Chandler Publishing Co., 1964), pp. 198-199.

17. Joseph Zubin, p. 395.

18. R.K. Freudenberg and J.P. Robertson, "Symptoms in Relation to Psychiatric Diagnosis and Treatment," *A.M.A. Archives of Neurological Psychiatry* 76 (1956): 14-22.

19. E. Zigler and L. Philips, "Psychiatric Diagnosis and Symptomatology," *Journal of Abnormal and Social Psychology* 63 (1961): 69-75.

20. M.M. Katz, F.O. Cole and H.A. Lowery, "Nonspecificity of Diagnosis of Paranoid Schizophrenia," *Archives of General Psychiatry* 11 (1964): 197-202.

21. Josephy Zubin, p. 389; and Joseph Zubin, L.D. Eron, and F. Schumer, *Experimental Approaches to Assessment of Behavior in Psychopathology* (New York: Wiley, 1965).

22. Joseph Zubin, p. 390.

23. A. Dershowitz, "Psychiatrists' Power in Civil Commitment," *Psychology Today* 2 (1969): 147.

24. E. Wenk, J. Robison, and G. Smith, "Can Violence Be Predicted?" *Crime and Delinquency* 18 (1972): 393-402.

25. H. Kozol, R. Boucher, and R. Garofalo, "The Diagnosis and Treatment of Dangerousness," *Crime and Delinquency* 18 (October 1972): 371-293.

26. Phil Standford, "Model 'Clockwork Orange' Prison—Patuxent Institution for Defective Delinquents," *New York Times Magazine* (Sept. 17, 1972): 9.

27. E. Megargee, "The Prediction of Violence with Psychological Tests," in C. Speilberger, ed., *Current Topics in Clinical and Community Psychology* (New York: The Academic Press, 1970), pp. 98-156.

28. Henry Steadmen and Joseph Cocozza, *Careers of the Criminally Insane: Excessive Social Control of Deviance* (Lexington, Mass: Lexington Books, 1974).

29. John Monahan, "The Prediction of Dangerousness," in D. Chappell and J. Monahan, eds. *Violence and Criminal Justice* (Lexington, Mass.: D.C. Heath & Co., 1975), pp. 15-32.

30. Jeff Coulter, *The Operations of Mental Health Personnel in an Urban Area* (Manchester, England: University of Manchester, unpublished dissertation, 1975), p. 28.

31. Thomas J. Scheff, pp. 175-176.

32. Ibid., pp. 182-184.

33. Ibid., pp. 155-168.

34. Thomas J. Scheff, *Mental Illness and the Social Processes* (New York: Harper and Row, 1967), p. 6.

35. David Mechanic, "Some Factors in Identifying and Defining Mental Illness," in S. Spitzer and N. Denzin, eds., *The Mental Patient: Studies in the Sociology of Deviance* (New York: McGraw-Hill Book Co., 1968), pp. 197-198.

36. Thomas J. Scheff, *Mental Illness,* pp. 113-117. Scheff argues against these two assumptions. According to Scheff, the first ignores key literature suggesting both the social nature of psychiatric disorders and the fact that unorganized or undiagnosed "mental illness" often dissipates without psychiatric intervention. The weakness of the second argument is suggested by the concept of "secondary deviance" and by the differential social outcomes afforded one stigmatized with the label of "being mentally ill."

37. Ennis and Litwack, pp. 720-732.

38. John Monahan, pp. 20-25.

39. The terms "more rational" or "idealized rationality" indicate a heavy emphasis on a "means-end" approach to social reality and thus are related to the ideal-type rationality discussed by Weber.

40. In this sense the critiques of the rationality of psychiatric decision-making parallel various sociologies of formal organization and/or bureaucracy which depict the informal rules that deflect or distort a reified "means-end" model of organizational activity. The informal processes are understood to compromise the formal rules and thus debunk the notion that the bureaucracies actually follow a model of idealized rationality. On paper (or in the table of organization) bureaucracies appear to be "rational" goal-obtaining entities. Upon a closer sociological analysis, however, they are revealed to be a considerably "nonrational" collection of competing subgroups—intramural status systems as well as instrumental needs.

The above "finding" does not appear to lessen the "should-be-more-rational" commitments of many students of formal organization. What is needed are mechanisms for minimizing the distortive impact of the "informal" variables (that is, "humanize" channels of communication, increase job satisfaction, institute participatory management styles, etc.). This approach preserves the image of idealized rationality in bureaucracy by neutralizing the effect of social forces which distort it.

41. Joseph Zubin, "Cross-National Study of Diagnosis of the Mental Disorders: Methodology and Planning," *American Journal of Psychiatry,* 125, 10 (April Supplement): 12-20.

42. L. Phillips and J.G. Draguns, "Classification of the Behavioral Disorders."

43. Harold Garfinkel, "The Rational Properties of Scientific and Common Sense Activities," *Studies in Ethnomethodology* (Englewood Cliffs, N.J.: Prentice-Hall, 1967), p. 263.

44. Jeff Coulter, p. 30.

45. Alfred Schutz, "The Problem of Rationality in the Social World," *Collected Papers II: Studies in Social Theory* (The Hague: Martinus Nijhoff, 1971), pp. 64-90.

46. Abraham Kaplan, pp. 3-11.

# 3

# Conceiving the Study: Labeling Theory, Ethnomethodology, and the Production of Psychiatric Accounts

*The distinctive character of the social reaction perspective . . . leads . . . to a consideration of how deviants come to be differentiated by imputations made about them by others, how these imputations activate systems of social control, and how those control activities become legitimated as institutional responses to deviance.*

John Kituse, "The 'New Conception of Deviance' and Its Critics"[1]

A concern with the procedures by which diagnosticians construct psychiatric assessments places the present study within the framework of the social reaction perspective on deviance. This chapter classifies the conceptual basis for this investigation by relating its theoretical interests to two traditions within the social reaction perspective: labeling theory and ethnomethodology. In the following pages we shall distinguish between these traditions, review the current debate over the adequacy of the labeling tradition, and make a case for adopting the ethnomethodological tradition as that most compatible with the issues raised by our own investigation.

At the same time we shall suggest the need to expand or modify the ethnomethodological framework so as to attend to certain issues (that is, power and social interests) which have received little explicit consideration in prior ethnomethodological research. The chapter closes with a statement of basic, theoretical commitments involved in considering psychiatric decision-making as a practical accomplishment of professional agents of social control.

## The Societal Reaction Perspective

The origins of the societal reaction perspective are often traced to Tannenbaum's discussion of the process and implications of "tagging" deviants.[2] Nonetheless, the conceptual framework of this perspective is clearly anticipated in Mead's consideration of the ritualistic drama of the criminal law. For Mead, the "majesty of the law," the "solemnity of the criminal court," and the "severity of the penal sanction" combined symbolically to inhibit rebellion by

31

law-abiding citizens, while dramatically signifying an outsider or stigmatized identity for those who are removed from the community by the social organization of punitive justice.[3]

The focus on the "creation" of deviance or outsider status in the process of public or social reaction was most explicitly stated by Becker. According to Becker's formulation, "deviance is *not* a quality of the act the person commits, but rather a consequence of the application by others of rules and sanctions to an "offender.' The deviant is one to whom that label has successfully been applied; deviant behavior is behavior that people so label."[4] Lemert expanded this notion by introducing the concept of "secondary deviance."[5] This idea considered the impact of "stigmatizing" social reaction in solidifying the outsider's identity for those initially labeled as deviants.

The work within the societal reaction perspective described to this point has loosely been referred to as labeling theory. It shifted substantive sociological inquiry away from a nearly exclusive concern with the sociocultural conditions that are likely to produce deviant behavior. It inquired, instead, into the process by which an individual or group is set apart as deviant and on the consequences of this singling-out process for those labeled and those doing the labeling. Methodologically this work challenged the basis of much etiological research by undermining the assumptions that all officially designated deviants "have actually committed a deviant act" and that "the category of those labeled deviant will contain all those who actually have broken a rule."[6] As suggested by the research reviewed in the previous chapter, some persons might be labeled deviant simply by the biases or perceptual error of official labelers. On the other hand, many rule violators "may escape apprehension and thus fail to be included in the population of 'deviants.' "[7] What then do those labeled as deviants have in common? The answer, according to Becker and others associated with the labeling tradition, is that "they share the label and experience of being labeled as outsiders."[8] Deviance is thus viewed as the product of interaction between those doing labeling and those who are targets of this process of social control.

### A Labeling Theory of Mental Illness

The most direct application of labeling theory to mental illness is found in the work of Scheff.[9] From his own research and from a review of the work of others, Scheff delineates nine propositions related to the social dimensions of mental illness. In the previous chapter we reviewed Scheff's conception of unlabeled mentally disordered behaviors as "residual deviance." We also considered Scheff's suggestion that certain organizational, ideological, financial, and political contingencies channel "residually deviant" behaviors into the category of "being mentally ill." In developing his formal proposition, Scheff contends that:

1. Residual rule-breaking arises from fundamentally diverse sources.
2. Relative to the rate of treated mental illness, the rate of unrecorded rule-breaking is extremely high.
3. Most residual rule-breaking is "denied" and is of transitory significance.
4. Stereotyped imagery of mental disorder is learned in early childhood.
5. The stereotypes of insanity are continually reaffirmed, inadvertently, in ordinary social interaction.
6. Labeled deviants may be rewarded for playing the stereotyped role.
7. Labeled deviants are punished when they attempt to return to conventional roles.
8. In a crisis occurring when a residual rule-breaker is publicly labeled, the deviant is highly suggestible and may accept the proffered role of the insane as the only alternative.
9. Among residual rule-breakers, labeling is the single most important cause of careers of residual deviants.

The first eight of Scheff's propositions assume that without labeling most residual deviance will not lead to a deviant career in madness or mental illness.[10] This assumption is made explicit in his final proposition. According to the ninth proposition, labeling is the focal point for understanding mentally ill behaviors. Nonetheless the importance of labeling is said to be itself contingent on seven additional variables. These include the degree of rule-breaking, the amount of rule-breaking, the visibility of rule-breaking, the power of the rule-breaker, the social distance between the rule-breaker and agents of social control, the tolerance level of a given community, and the cultural availability of alternative nondeviant roles. The first two variables, degree and amount of rule-breaking, are characteristics of the individual and his or her behavior. The last five variables are said to represent elements of the social system which are independent of a particular behavioral display of residual rule-breaking. The logic of Scheff's position regarding the preeminence of labeling as "the single most important cause of a career of residual deviance" is that the last five variables will have more impact on the recognition of and reaction to "mental illness" than will the first two variables. In other words, social contingencies, independent of individually "bizarre" behaviors, are proposed as being more significant than the behaviors themselves in the determination that an individual is mentally ill.

The core of Scheff's "labeling theory" (his ninth proposition) is tested in a two-phase study of official psychiatric decision-making.[11] The first phase (obtaining independent psychiatric ratings on potential candidates for involuntary hospitalization) revealed high levels of clinical uncertainty as to whether labeling targets were "actually" dangerous or disturbed enough to satisfy state standards for involuntary commitment. Despite such uncertainty, the study's second phase (observations of the five-stage legal commitment process) found that in a sample of 116 consecutive commitment proceedings, and in an additional sample of eighty court records reviewed, there was not a single recommendation for release. These findings led to Scheff's observation concerning a psychiatric "presumption of illness" and to his analysis of the impact of social variables discussed in the previous chapter. Overall, Scheff concludes that his work provides clear documentary support for the labeling theory of mental illness.

### Critiques of Labeling Theory

Despite the seeming clarity of its intent, both theoretical and empirical adequacy of labeling theory have been subjects for considerable criticism in recent years. Empirical critiques have been rendered in a number of substantive areas (for example, delinquency, criminality, and mental retardation).[12] They have been nowhere more forceful, however, than on the topic of mental illness. The leading critic in this area has been Gove, whose review of the "available evidence . . . indicates that the social reaction formulation of how a person becomes mentally ill is substantially incorrect."[13] Gove, however, often appears to misunderstand the attempt of labeling theorists to offer simply another perspective on mental illness, rather than to represent a new causal explanation for the phenomenon as a whole. Despite the fact that the major proponents of the labeling position have argued that their work represents more of a "sensitizing perspective" than a causal explanation,[14] Gove charges that "virtually all labeling theorists seem to hold that their perspective is a powerful explanatory tool when applied to mental illness."[15] Gove is inconsistent in his characterization of the intent of labeling theory. Elsewhere he acknowledges that the labeling position is a "sensitizing theory or general perspective," but argues that his purpose is to "state this sensitizing theory in such a way that it can be empirically evaluated."[16] The results of Gove's "tests" and Scheff's "rebuttals" are well known to those familiar with the recent Gove-Scheff exchange in the *American Sociological Review.*

Citing a variety of studies, Gove's criticisms appear to fall into four general categories. His first criticism appears to be directed at Scheff's first proposition (that is, residual rule-breaking arises from fundamentally diverse sources). In contradiction to what he believes to be the position of labeling theory, Gove argues that persons who are reacted to as mentally ill are in fact mentally ill. Their behavior, in other words, is truly abnormal or disturbed. This argument is buttressed by three sources of evidence. The first is based upon studies which compare the scores of psychiatric patients and controls on a variety of scales which measure psychiatric symptomatology (HOS Scale, Langner Scale, Gurin Scale, Lubin Depression Checklist, etc.). A general finding of these studies is "that persons in psychiatric treatment are more likely to manifest psychiatric symptoms that those not in treatment."[17] The second source of evidence cited by Gove concerns research revealing that "persons hospitalized for mental illness are much more likely than comparable controls to have experienced a critical life event just prior to their hospitalization."[18] The third describes studies which suggest that "for the two most serious forms of mental illness, schizophrenia and manic-depressive psychosis, there appears to be a very strong genetic component to the disorders."[19] In the thinking of Gove, these findings support the psychiatric theory and undermine labeling theory. They reportedly show that "persons who receive psychiatric treatment are mentally ill and . . . manifest more psychiatric symptoms than those not receiving such treatment. In contrast, the societal reaction suggests that persons receiving psychiatric treatment do not have an underlying psychiatric disorder."[20]

Gove's second argument suggests that the informal tolerance of friends, relatives, and acquaintances are as important or more important in deciding upon mental illness than are official labeling processes. A large part of Gove's reasoning is based on a pioneering study by Yarrow et al. which suggested that wives of disturbed husbands utilize a variety of denial and coping mechanisms to keep their spouses in the community (and out of the official labeling process) until the behavior of the husband becomes intolerable or impossible to deal with.[21] Other studies which reveal the gross disturbance or havoc created by patients prior to hospitalization are also cited as documentation of the exaggerated claims of labeling theory.[22] (This line of argumentation appears to be directed against the third of Scheff's propositions concerning the transitory nature of residual rule-breaking.)

The third of Gove's criticisms is aimed at Scheff's ninth proposition, which concerns the singular significance of labeling as a cause of careers for the mentally ill. Gove argues that a consideration of voluntary admissions, the official screening process, and variables related to status and power reflect poorly on the labeling position. With regard to voluntary admissions, Gove suggests that "from the societal reaction perspective, it is very hard to see why persons would voluntarily stigmatize themselves by seeking psychiatric treatment, particularly when it involved inpatient care."[23] He argues that two studies which do report on voluntary admissions reveal high rates of "screening" away patients. Gove does not mention, however, that these studies also reveal that key social variables have a significant impact on this process of screening.[24]

A selectivity of evidence also appears to characterize Gove's discussion of the official screening process. A study by Bittner on police encounters with the allegedly mentally disturbed, unpublished manuscripts by Tucker regarding the actions of psychiatrists to recommend commitment, and research by Wilde which found a psychiatric screening agency approved requests for commitment in only 33 percent of the cases are all cited as evidence that "officials do not assume illness, but, in fact, proceed rather cautiously, screening out a substantial number of persons."[25] Yet, Bittner's observations that police "avail themselves of various forms of denial,"[26] Tucker's finding "that there was a correlation between the police officer labeling a person 'demented' and [psychiatric] disposition,"[27] and Wilde's discovery of a 98 percent commitment request approval rate for hospital psychiatrists[28] would seemingly also support the "social contingencies" position of labeling theory. The importance of recognizing this selectivity on Gove's part is magnified by the manner in which he interprets studies on the later phases of the screening process. Gove acknowledges that studies of psychiatric examinations and court hearings generally reflect very high rates of commitment recommendations and decisions. He reasons, however, that by virtue of substantial screening it is quite possible that by the time of the hearing most prospective patients do indeed have a serious disorder. Gove uses similar reasoning to reinterpret what might otherwise pass as social contingencies affecting the commitment decision process. For instance, where Miller and Schwartz note the differential impact of a patient's "in-court" resistance,[29] Gove alternatively suggests that nonresisters may have been "in fact" more disordered than those who resisted.[30]

Gove's discussion of social position and power is also intended to underscore the inadequacy of labeling theory. Regarding the sociometric position of the labeled mentally ill, research is cited which shows that more powerful persons (occupying critical positions in the family) are more likely to be quickly hospitalized.[31] Labeling theory, contends Gove, would predict the opposite (that is, that the less powerful are more vulnerable to labeling by others). Gove's analysis of class differentials in rates of mental illness similarly suggests a reversal of the basic tenets of the labeling position. He admits that, on first glance, various epidemiological literature (showing that lower-class individuals are more likely to be treated as mentally ill) seems supportive of the labeling position. Another interpretation of these differentials, however, is said to be found in "traditional psychiatric explanations [which] see stress as more common in the lower class, and those that would also predict higher rates of mental illness in the lower class."[32] Gove marshals four lines of evidence to support this latter interpretation. This evidence includes: (1) the results of various community surveys which are said to document higher rates of mental illness among the lower classes;[33] (2) research suggesting that "members of the lower class tend to see only a narrow range of aggressive, antisocial behavior as creating a need for psychiatric treatment, whereas persons in the middle and upper class perceive a much wider range of psychopathological behavior as indicating a need for psychiatric care";[34] (3) research suggesting that lower-class individuals delay requests for treatment (even when needed);[35] and (4) literature revealing the more serious (disorganized and violent) symptomatology of lower-class individuals.[36] Taken as a whole, these findings are said to support the psychiatric position and to deemphasize labeling theory.

Other "power" variables are also believed to point out the flaws in the labeling position. Studies of marital status reveal that lack of social resources (not being married) was associated with a delay in seeking psychiatric treatment.[37] Studies also show that (less powerful) blacks are not overrepresented (as the victims of labeling) among hospitalized patients.[38] These findings are taken as contradictions to labeling theory. The fact that women, considered to have relatively low social status, were overrepresented among patients was not taken as evidence in support of labeling. Instead, it is argued that community studies show that women in our society "really" do have higher rates of mental illness, while this was not the case prior to World War II, and is not the case in nonindustrialized societies.[39] Furthermore, the social reaction to mental illness among relatively more powerful men (when compared to women) is more severe and is characterized by prompter and lengthier psychiatric intervention.[40] Here, as in other cases, labeling is not seen as the most significant factor causing a career of mental illness.

Gove's final criticism of labeling theory focuses on Scheff's seventh proposition, that labeled deviants are punished when they attempt to return to conventional roles. Scheff's original formulation relied heavily on the "rejection" findings of Phillips. It is noted that subsequent work by this same author indicated that rejection was more strongly associated with the degree of disturbed behavior than with the supposedly stigmatizing source of help.[41] Other work suggests that ex-patients do not perceive the hospitalization experience in terms of long-term stigmatization and that more ex-patients were employed one year after hospitalization than were in the period prior to being hospitalized.[42] Elsewhere it is argued that the "psychopharmacological revolution" and the introduction of "new psychotherapeutic techniques" have led to shorter stays for patients and to a sharp decline in the number of persons in the role of the chronically mentally ill.[43] This is, of course, believed to neutralize the impact of hospitalization on so-called secondary deviance. Furthermore, studies are cited in relation to psychiatric recidivism in which hospital "returnees were decidely sicker than the community patients" and would indicate "that intrinsic features of the illness are of greater consequence in precipitating readmission than are the variations in the way significant others perceive, evaluate, or tolerate mental illness."[44] Again, the predictions of labeling theory are interpreted as inadequate or inoperative. In summary, Gove suggests that the weight of existing evidence favors the psychiatric perspective over that of labeling theory.

Gove's conclusions about labeling theory are stated as if a choice has to be made between perspectives in deciding on a model which most adequately explains the phenomenon of mental illness. As he states the issue, "[T]he question should be which perspective is most consistent with and best accounts for the majority of the available evidence? . . . [I]t is very clear that if we . . . choose between the psychiatric perspective and the labeling perspective, the evidence overwhelmingly supports the psychiatric perspective."[45] Does it?

It should be noted that Gove's criticisms appear to address only four (though admittedly the most important) of Scheff's original nine propositions.

More important is the fact that Scheff returns to the debate, arguing against a number of Gove's substantive and methodological claims.[46] Regarding Gove's first objection (and in defense of his own first proposition), Scheff's contention is that labeling theory never denied the possibility that residual deviance could arise out of such traditional psychiatric sources as stress, critical life events, and genetic or physiological disturbances. Indeed, Scheff's earlier work had acknowledged that "it has been demonstrated repeatedly that particular cases of mental disorder had their origin in genetic, bio-chemical, or physiological conditions." What Scheff appears to be saying is that the origins, causes, or etiology of certain behaviors are not at issue in a test of labeling. What are at issue are the processes that categorize, name, tag, or label this behavior as "bizarre," "really mentally ill," "prophetic," or whatever. A return to Scheff's previous anthropological examples concerning the differential labeling of overtly similar behavior would seemingly offer both a clarification of his position and a defense of the propositions as originally formulated.

In response to Gove's criticisms of his third proposition (regarding the transitory nature of residual deviance) Scheff scores the methodological inadequacy of work like that of Yarrow et al., which obtains information on incidents of serious disruptive behavior solely by reports of family members. If one accepts the conclusions of Laing and Esterson (which Scheff does) regarding the frequent etiology of mental disorders in distortive communication networks, then one should approach with caution research which simply asks possible victimizers to explain the problems of their victim. Scheff's rebuttal would have been even stronger had he suggested (which he did not) that his original proposition emphasized that residual deviance is "denied" as well as "transitory." After all, a focus on "denial mechanisms" is a key dimension of the studies which Gove cites to undermine Scheff's position. In all fairness, however, it should be commented that these studies do appear to document the "experienced" (if not necessary) severity and nontransitory nature of behaviors that come to be labeled as mentally ill.

Regarding Gove's criticism of his major labeling proposition, Scheff clarifies and restates the findings of his original research and suggests that thirteen of eighteen studies, which directly attempt to test the "social contingencies" aspect of the theory, provide support for the labeling position. Scheff admits that the perfunctory nature of screening at later stages (that is, court hearings) could hypothetically result from previous screening away of all but the seriously impaired and/or dangerous. His own work, which gathered data in both early and late screening phases, is said, however, to deny such an interpretation. Moreover, Gove's suggestion that power and status differentials point to findings in the opposite direction from labeling theory is open to question on a number of counts. Remember that much of Gove's reasoning was based on findings of community surveys or ratings of symptomatology. These were said to reveal differential evidence for the existence of serious mental disorders between classes (and between men and women). These findings were taken as "fact" by Gove, despite the "fact" that numerous other studies reveal considerable perceptual "class-based biases" on the part of psychiatric raters.[47] Gove does not address or review these findings.

One could additionally question Gove's assumption that persons with more centralized family positions or who are married are more powerful (and should be hypothetically more resistant to labeling). Remember, it is not labeling theory which makes this assumption, but its critics. From one perspective such persons would seem to have more power or resources, but from another it seems likely that they also have more responsibilities and role obligations. In other words, it is possible that their social commitments make their bizarre behaviors more vulnerable to labeling, even though they may be rated as more powerful in accordance with other sociometric measures. All of this is not to say that each of Gove's criticisms is without a basis. His observations concerning differential rates of treatment-seeking and delays in treatment appear to support an argument that upper-middle-class persons may be under more pressure to seek some kind of official handling of their problems. Even Scheff recognizes the awkward overstatement of his original "most important single cause" position. Recently he has expressed regret over the use of this formulation, suggesting that the theoretical strength of his argument concerns the relative importance of social system, when compared to individualistic variables in the labeling process.[48]

In relation to Gove's final objection to the stigmatizing and "secondary deviance" propositions of labeling theory, Scheff admits "that existing evidence concerning stigma is weaker than [he] had expected it would be."[49] He nonetheless warns against an uncritical acceptance of the results of a revolution in psychotherapeutic drugs and treatment. He points to recent work which suggests that patients initially receiving tranquilizers respond better than those not receiving them, but that, in the long run, patients who do not get tranquilizers respond far better than those who do.[50] Scheff also argues that changes in mental health laws (in part inspired by the work of labeling theory) may be more associated with a decrease in the number of patients than is any revolution in treatment per se.[51] He concludes his rebuttal with the statement that "the purpose of a purely sociological model is not to replace the psychiatric perspective, but to serve as a corrective to the exclusive emphasis of the medical model on the isolated individual."[52]

### Labeling: A Distorted Debate and the Problem of Normativity

The discussion so far has focused on the debate over the empirical adequacy of labeling theory—its critique and its defense. This debate, however, has somewhat distorted the distinctive theoretical or substantive contribution of the societal reaction perspective. This distortion is intrinsic to Scheff's original formulation of the problem. It is not inherent in the societal reaction perspective itself.

Recall that labeling theory originally offered both a *new* theoretical perspective (a focus on the process of deviantizing) and a methodological argument against an *old* perspective (that all officially defined deviants are "really" deviants). Much of Scheff's work, explicitly and implicitly, is an attempt to advance this second offering. He suggests that a large percentage of persons who are not really residual deviants get classified as such anyway. As such, his work is typical of the "critical-reformer" perspective outlined in the previous chapter. It is Scheff's critique that Gove is actually criticizing. His arguments are geared toward showing that the *old* (psychiatric) perspective is not so bad after all, and that most persons who are classified as mentally ill are really ill. In this regard, both the critic and the defender appear to be operating under similar ontological assumptions. Both make a distinction between "objects," which are there (that is, crazy people, residual deviants, or the mentally ill), and "subjects," which recognize whether they are there or not. The difference between Gove and Scheff, at this level of their debates, is simply a difference in the degree to which various social systems' variables are understood to distort the accuracy by which "subjects" (official labelers) see whether "objects" (the potentially labeled) are "really" there or not. As such, the debate misses what is theoretically *new* in the social reaction perspective—an eradication of the subject-object distinction by attending to the process in which the "reality" of an individual's deviance is accomplished or created by the definitional work of others.

Perhaps the distortion described above is inevitable, given the inconsistent theoretical formulation of labeling theory. As Gibbs insightfully points out, labeling theory has shown considerable inconsistency regarding the problem of normativity.[53] Despite its repeated claim that there is no normatively recognizable or "objective" deviance aside from social reactions to it, its proponents have introduced such ambiguous constructs as "secret" or "undiscovered" deviance.[54] How, from the perspective of labeling theory, can something be described as deviant when it is secret, and, hence, not labeled? A similar problem arises regarding Scheff's concept of residual deviance. As with secret deviance, this concept seems to imply a normative recognition that a rule has been broken prior to a social reaction. Consider Scheff's discussion of norms or rules of conduct violated by residual deviants. Scheff employs the phrase "unnameable rule breaking" when describing the way that these "strange, bizarre and frightening persons" fail to fulfill even the simplest conversational rules (not facing the partner, not showing appropriate eye contact, not recognizing the expected spatial relations, etc.).[55] Through this terminology residual deviance is distinguished from other norm violations (such as crime, perversion, drunkenness, or bad manners) which are said to be more readily classifiable in terms of culturally available vocabularies. On the other hand, residual rule-breaking only becomes named when these violations "sometimes" lead to the labeling of the violator as mentally ill."[56]

Scheff's statement is conceptually ambiguous. Although it has no name, the residual rule-breaking apparently has been recognized as a violation of normative expectations before it is ever considered for labeling. Calling this form of rule-breaking "unnameable" or "residual" does little to clarify the issue.

Gibbs attempts to interject clarity at the point where the labeling formulation stumbles into confusion.[57] Why worry about the social reaction in defining deviance? It is only occasionally present anyway. It is only sometimes present with "residual deviance" and never present with "secret deviance." What is always present, and what precedes the process of labeling, is the violation of conduct rules or social norms. The problem, then, for the student of deviance is to specify those behaviors which are evaluated as rule-breaking or violating the norms in a given society.[58] Gibbs uses two examples to exemplify his argument. In the first he asks the reader to imagine two persons on the street. One is naked. The other is not. Need one wait to see how each is reacted to in order to decide which is the deviant? After all, won't one be immediately seen as in violation of a rather clear set of societal norms or rules? In his second example, Gibbs criticizes Becker's interpretation of a Trobriand marital dispute (reported by Malinowski) as an instance of the nominalistic ambiguity of labeling theory.[59] Becker suggests that the man who has sexual relations with his mother's sister does something which is generally disapproved. The act does not become deviant, however, until the woman's discarded lover returns and accuses (or labels) the violator. Why wait to focus on the accusal or labeling process, asks Gibbs. Hasn't the act already been evaluated as violating normative expectations? Implicitly, Malinowski, Becker, the discarded lover, and everyone else must have recognized that a norm or rule was broken. If not, how did they know that the accusal was an accusal? Preceding the accusal and the instigation of the labeling process was the evaluation of a norm violation or rule breach.

Gibbs's formulation is intriguing. He suggests that it explicates the element of normative evaluation implicit in labeling theory and in the psychiatric perspective.[60] According to Gibbs, labeling theory's attention to the problem of societal reaction and the psychiatric perspective's concern with abnormality both implicitly presuppose the fact that something has been evaluated as being wrong, as breaking the rules. Their debate, after all, is not over this issue, but over whether or not the evaluation was correct. At its extreme, labeling theory offers an account of the "incorrectness" of the mental illness ascription by suggesting that an actor's rule-breaking is a product of victimization by a bad social environment.[61] Rule violators are converted into victims. At the other extreme, the psychiatric perspective accounts for the "correctness" of a mental illness diagnosis by suggesting that an actor's rule-breaking is the disturbed product of a psychiatric pathology. Rule violators are converted into patients.

While Gibbs is helpful in delineating conceptual inconsistencies in the labeling and psychiatric perspectives, his own formulation is no easy solution to the study of deviance. His preference for defining deviance "by reference to norms" confronts him with the problem of identifying the rules which spell out the dos and don'ts of normative behavior. According to Kituse, the sociologist addressing this problem has but two solutions: to survey members of the social system as to their expectations of others or to infer rules from observations of how members actually behave.[62]

As solutions, however, these two alternatives present further problems. Verbal statements may be what members say but they are no assurance that they are what they do. Furthermore, such "statements may not even be 'normative' in the sense that they urge that persons *ought* to behave as their statements specify, but simply represent what is said when people are asked about conduct in certain circumstances, an expression of an ideal that prescribes no sanctions when the norm is violated, set aside, or otherwise ignored."[63]

Inferring norms from behavior may be even more complicated. Since a multiplicity of inferences may be possible, given a particular observation, the sociologist is confronted with the task of constructing valid rules of inference. These observer rules imply a "correspondence" or "matching theory" of knowledge, in which it is never doubted that there really are norms out there.[64] The problem is to decide upon a set of operational definitions which best represent the normative world as it really exists. It should not be surprising if this problem resembles the debate between labeling theory and the psychiatric perspective over which sets of definitions best "fit" the phenomenon as it really is. As Gibbs has demonstrated, both of these perspectives are implicitly committed to the concept of normativity, and, hence, also to a matching or corresponding theory of knowledge.[65]

Decisions regarding adequate operational definitions of norms and norm violations are no simple matter. Such definitions entail a high degree of specificity regarding the questions of what conduct is prescribed or proscribed, by whom, for whom, in what situations, under what circumstances, assuming what degree of mental and social competence, etc. Moreover, it may be argued that sociologists have not been very successful in specifying all these variables for all or even most situations. Instead, "the common practice is for the sociologist to gloss over the methodological problems by relying, as a [presumed] member of the system being studied, on his or her own implicit and tactly held understanding of social norms."[66]

The sociological glossing described above is particularly troublesome for two reasons. First, it ignores the fact their social backgrounds, training, and political ideologies hardly qualify sociologists as "typical members" of a cultural system. As Kituse states, "Sociologists may find that members ignore, dismiss, and even applaud those acts that sociologists classify as unambiguously clear violations of the norm."[67] An interesting example of this point is provided in a study by

Gorgoff on how prison inmates interpret their own behavior.[68] In this project, researchers were trained to type inmate behavior according to Merton's "means-ends" scheme of deviance. Sociological observers had no problem in recognizing that most inmates were acting as "conformists" in obeying prison norms. A consultation of the perspectives of inmates on this matter, however, revealed that many who overtly acted "as if" they conformed were in actuality "ritualists" who simply played out typically expedient means so as to get out quicker. What was inferred as conformity by the observers was actually deviance from the actor's perspective.

The second problem with sociological glossing is that it ignores the situated character of deviance. For instance, "the naked and nonnaked persons on the street" example offered by Gibbs is transformed into an entirely different interpretation when we realize that the street is in the middle of a nudist camp. Gibbs's question (Won't one be immediately seen as in violation of a rather clear set of societal norms or rules?) is presented in a different light. The evaluation of normativity becomes less "immediate" and more "problematic." It is understood to be preceded by a certain amount of definitional or judgmental work (by the work of social reaction). It is this work, involved in the situated constitution of deviance, that is at the heart of the societal reaction perspective.

Consider as another example of the situated character of deviance Scheff's depiction of the normative rules governing the display of appropriate interactional behavior. These (roughly) include: (1) when holding a conversation, face your interlocutor; (2) when gazing at your interlocutor, look toward his eyes, not his forehead, etc.; (3) when engaging an interlocutor, do so at an easy speaking distance, neither one inch away nor across the room. The regular violation of these rules, suggests Scheff, can lead to the ascriptive label of being mentally ill. Yet, as Coulter points out, this ascriptive process is considerably more complex in everyday life. By no means can it be said that every violation of Scheff's interactional rules leads to the labeling of mental illness. Depending on the situated character of the observer-observed interaction a person not facing his interlocutor may be seen to be confiding a secret, talking idly, being preoccupied with private thoughts, or even being a shifty character. Each possible interpretation represents a situated alternative to the recognition that one is being mentally ill. So too with "incorrect" gazing (as in the "insulting stare") and inappropriate distancing (as in the joking breach or intimate reduction of typical spatial arrangements).[69]

Given the contextual or situated variation of rule-breaking and norm violation, where should the sociologist turn? Should an attempt be made to specify all known contextual contingencies and attach them to Scheff's or anyone else's theory of deviance? Coulter thinks not. He suggests that "there cannot be a codifiable totality of social circumstances in the sense in which there are codifiable (*and manipulable*) 'conditions of occurrence' in physics and chemistry. Contextual particulars," he continues, "cannot stand as sociological analogues to the physicist's conditions-of-occurrence of some natural events."[70] The best such an analogue could do would be to specify probabilities for recognized norm violations given this and that circumstance. This approach, however, would by-pass the everyday process whereby actors assess action-in-context and decide on the appropriateness of norms that provide a reasonable account of what is happening (or is not but should be happening). In other words, I am suggesting that rather than existing "out there" prior to the scene of social interaction, norms arise in, are a product of, and are used to provide accounts for the structure of social interaction. As Coulter states the issue, "Members do not routinely appraise conduct in terms solely of its conformity to or deviation from some stipulated standard of competent activity [*a package of preexisting norms and rules*]; they appraise conduct-in-context."[71]

If norm violations are the products of actors' judgmental work and not mere behaviors, then to appreciate fully the problem of deviance the sociologist must turn his or her attention away from a catalogue of potential norms and norm violations to the contextbound cataloging work of actors themselves. Actors' accounting practices (that is, decisions as to whether perceived actions are excused or inexcusable, justified or unjustifiable, etc.) become the focal point for a study of deviance. Sociologists are freed from the dilemma of trying to decide whether their definitions or those of social actors (members) are a more appropriate operationalization of norm violations. According to Kituse, "Definitions ... of members ... must prevail, however 'misinformed,' 'erroneous,' or 'misguided' they may appear to be from the sociologist's standpoint. The alternative of invoking the sociologist's definitions as the standard for assessing normative behavior, is to face the problem of accounting, on the one hand, for the failure of members to negatively sanction behavior that is 'obviously deviant,' and on the other for the imposition of such sanctions in the absence of 'norm violating' behavior."[72] It is this focus on members' accounting practices, on the interactional, contextbound process of deviant attribution, which is offered as something *distinctive* or *new* by the social reaction perspective. It is free of assumptions about preexisting norms and rules and thus frees the researcher to investigate the construction, use, and consequences of norms and rules in the process of day-to-day social interaction.

### Ethnomethodology: An Alternative Formulation of the Social Reaction Perspective

The focus on the process of deviant attribution has always been a substantive concern of the societal reaction perspective since its formuation by Becker and Lemert. This concern has emerged as particularly explicit in major papers by Erikson, Kituse, and Goode,[73] but has often been distorted by a methodologically based debate with advocates of an "objectivist perspective" over the "correctness" of certain deviant attributions. The "correctness issue" has side-tracked labeling theory by tying it to an inconsistent assumption regarding preexisting normativity. Such ambiguous conceptions as "secret deviance" and "residual deviance" appear to presume some evaluation of rule breach or norm violation prior to the process of labeling. Moreover, Scheff's arguments concerning the correctness and reliability of behavior labels appear to presume some implicit standard of "real" deviance or normativity independent of the definitional work of labeling agents.

While labeling theory has been sidetracked by the issue of implicit normativity, another strand or tradition within the societal reaction framework has not. This strand, originating in the works of Harold Garfinkel, is referred to as ethnomethodology.[74] It concerns itself with the methods or practices that everyday actors employ to accomplish a "reasonable account" of what is happening in social interaction and to provide a "sense of structure" for the interaction itself.[75] For ethnomethodology, normativity (or the sense of things being rule-governed) is conceived of as a production rather than as a presumption. It is the result of the interpretive work that Garfinkel alternately refers to as "accounting practices" or "the activities of practical reasoning,"[76] and which Cicourel has designated, at various times, as "interpretive procedures, interpretive strategies," or "basic interpretive rules."[77] No matter what this work is called it basically refers to the range of descriptive language or gestural practices that actors employ, in the context of concrete social interaction, in order to produce a sense of social life as structured. A number of these practices (doing the practices of "reciprocity of perspectives," of "et cetera," of "creating normal forms," and so on) have been described and enumerated in the ethnomethodological literature.[78] Their relationship to the study of deviance may best be understood, however, by reference to three of their constitutive elements: the principles of indexicality, reflexivity, and documentary interpretation.

According to the ethnomethodological perspective, the structuring of an event, by rendering an account of it as deviance, is not done by checking to see if some rule or norm "out there" was broken. It is done, rather, by a member's active interpretive work, situated within the boundaries of a particular context, such that the context and the work within it are said to mutually determine each other. This mutual determination of work and context is referred to as the principle of indexicality. It suggests that the recognition or attribution of deviance (or anything else) is inherently bound to the context of its presentation and production. As Garfinkel suggests, "The objectivity of accounts are not independent of the socially organized occasion of their use."[79]

A second principle of ethnomethodology of particular importance for the study of deviance is that of reflexivity. By reflexivity we simply refer to the manner in which actors' interpretive accounts (verbal or nonverbal) come to alter the setting (or, in Garfinkel's terms, become constitutive features of the settings) in which they are employed. In other words, interpretive accounts are not only bound by the context in which the occur (indexically), but through their very expression they create new contexts and thereby become a part of the phenomenon which they seek to render meaningful (reflexively).

A further dimension of reflexivity in most everyday social interaction is its relative unnoticeability. By unnoticed reflexivity we refer to that property of everyday account-rendering by which reflexivity itself becomes "uninteresting" or taken for granted and for all practical purposes dropped from consideration in favor of that which it served to produce—a sense of the world as given in this or that way.[80] On the other hand, to notice reflexivity would call into question the existence of the world independent of my own contextbound interpretive work, which in turn may question the basis for the questioning (itself a product of being reflexive about reflexivity, etc., etc., etc.). While this problem may lead the student of reflexivity or reflexive interpretive work down what some have called the path of "infinite regress,"[81] it is a problem that the successful development of "unnoticed reflexivity" spares most actors in everyday life. The unnoticed character of reflexivity suggests that once members' interpretive work has accomplished a "reasonably accountable sense of structure," it loses the character of having been work and becomes experienced as an objectified element of the context in which working was done. In other words, that which is produced in the process of work is then experienced as having existed "out there" prior to and independent of the work. It takes on the appearance of being real (or governed by rules outside oneself). This appearance is thus experienced as independent of the production process in which it arose. Experientially the actor switches from the mode of being a creator to that of being a discoverer. Something is experienced as deviant not just because that is the way I have come to see it, but because I have discovered that is the way it is.

The sense of discovering norm violations does not negate the fact that the "sense of discovery" is, itself, a "reflexive" product of the process in which deviance is created.[82] Somewhat paradoxically the successful end-product of doing the work of creating deviance is to "forget" (or at least be inattentive to) the fact that any work was even involved. This reflexive disguising of the created character of deviance is discussed by Melvin Pollner, who suggests that even though deviance is a product of a community's response to its own needs for social control, an integral feature of this deviantizing is that the deviance itself will be seen as entirely independent of the response pattern which defines it. According to Pollner, "While a community creates deviance, it may simultaneously mask its creative work from itself."[83]

The method of documentary interpretation is a third element of ethnomethodology of relevance to the phenomenon of social deviance. Garfinkel borrows the term documentary interpretation from Mannheim. It refers to the method that both everyday actors and social scientists use to identify meaningful action patterns behind the appearance of mere behavioral stimuli.

Appearances are treated as but a document or expression of some underlying pattern.[84] According to Garfinkel, "Not only is the underlying pattern derived from its individual documentary evidences, but the individual documentary evidences, in their turn, are interpreted on the basis of 'what is known' about the underlying pattern. Each is used to elaborate the other."[85]

Of particular significance for deviance is the suggestion that the rules (by which an actor is judged as in compliance or violation of a normative order) are seen as the patterned product of this method of documentary interpretation. This is not to say that rules or norms do not exist. It is to say that they exist only as the end-product of the judgmental work by which actors size up a situation, interpret it as an instance of a more general pattern, and then use the general pattern as a device for giving order to what they perceive or experience in the present. Rules are not assumed to exist independently of the documentary work of actors. Working with rules, actors produce a structured definition of a particular situation. "Rules, like actors and situations, do not appear except in a web of practical circumstances. Intertwined, the actor, rules, and the present definition of the situation constitute the situation. No single one of these can be abstracted out and treated as either cause or effect."[86]

Taken together the principles of indexicality, reflexivity, and documentary interpretation illustrate the ethnomethodological claim that all rules or norms are essentially open or empty until they are filled in by the contextbound interpretive work of actors, wherein appearances are treated as patterns which are (reflexively) recognized as having a life of their own. According to ethnomethodologists Mehan and Wood, "Without this work, a rule has no meaning, no life at all."[87] With this work, actors produce a sense of normativity: the ordered appearance that their actions are guided by or in violation of rules or norms outside themselves.

### The Conceptual Framework of the Present Study:
### The Production of Psychiatric Definitions

The ethnomethodological perspective discards the implicit assumption of normativity. It focuses, instead, on the explicit production of a sense of normativity. Thus, when contrasted to labeling theory, it offers a more consistent conceptual structure for the societal reaction perspective on deviance. The "correctness" issue (whether an attribution of deviance is accurate or not) becomes a non-issue. In the case of mental illness, the debate over the adequacy of the societal reaction perspective shifts away from attempts to determine which model (the medical or labeling) "best accounts for the majority of the available evidence."[88] The ethnomethodological perspective is not concerned about whether a label is correct or valid. It is concerned about the nature of the necessary process of interaction between agents of control and targets of labeling. It is through this interaction that an imputation of deviance emerges, is defended, and is rationalized as reflecting a reality independent of its imputer. As Kituse argues, "The contention is not that agents of control act without regard to the behavior of the one labeled, but that in labeling, rule breaking behavior is imputed by others to the deviant."[89]

The "fact" that many prospective mental patients may have been disturbed for some time prior to hospitalization may seem to challenge labeling theory. It does not negate the central proposition of the ethnomethodological strand within the societal reaction perspective. The control issue remains the process by which imputations of deviance are constructed and applied. Hence, "facts," such as a history of disturbed behavior, are not evaluated as to their validity. The ethnomethodologist does not argue that deviance was "really" not where labelers imputed it to be. Instead the "facts" of deviance are treated as productions (or "artifacts") through which deviance may be simultaneously understood as a creation (by labeling actors) and as a reality (independent of labeling actors). In other words, the constitution of the "facts of deviance," rather than their evaluation, is at the core of the ethnomethodological approach. The question of whether something is "really"deviant is suspended in favor of a study of the process by which deviance is recognized as "real."

The present research has selected the ethnomethodological perspective as its primary conceptual framework because this perspective allows the researcher to appreciate most fully the detailed interactional work that actors perform in generating an attribution of deviance. Rather than evaluating the validity of diagnostic attributions, it seeks to study the indexical, documentary, and reflexive work which generates and sustains psychiatric decisions.

## Theoretical Commitments

The present analysis is guided by an ethnomethodological perspective on deviance. It is thus not concerned with the "objective" accuracy of attributions of deviance. It is concerned with the interactional methods by which agents of social control privately name, publicly designate, and professionally account for the deviance of others. Our theoretical commitments are summarized in the following statement. (This statement of theoretical commitments contains five analytic assumptions. Each will be examined in turn.)

*Diagnostic agents work to accomplish a "sense of structure," by naming patients as types of persons, in accordance with their own perceived interests and in relation to the resistance of others.*

*Diagnostic Agents*

In examining diagnostic agents we are concerned with the operations of a particular type of social actor—the imputational specialist. As mentioned at the
onset of this book, modern society relies upon this type of "expert" actor (the
judge, the police officer, the psychiatric professional) to determine whether
a suspected individual is "really deviant." As Lofland points out, the person on
the street, immersed in conventional pursuits, has too little time, interest, or
believed skill to act as an effective coder of deviance. Moreover, it is argued
that a regular flow of deviant imputations (and hence the boundaries of social
control) can be easily facilitated by paying persons to spend a major portion
of their time making such decisions—by professionalizing the task of discovering
deviance.[90]

Clearly, the Lima court order assumed the need for such imputational
specialists, expertly competent "to discover 'out there' in the empirical world
those sorts of people they have been trained to see."[91] It is the methods and
imputational procedures of this specialized type of social actor that we are
committed to explore and to explicate.

*Work*

Diagnostic work is conceived of as involving a three-stage process, which is believed to be informed at all times by the principles of indexicality, documentary
interpretation, and reflexivity.[92] The three work stages include the development
of diagnostic types, the designation of these types, and the renegotiation of
types.

The first stage in this process involves the interpretive or cognitive work of
an individual in typing or categorizing a patient as this or that kind of person.
For our purposes, we are concerned with the work which types and categorizes
an individual as mentally ill or dangerous or in need of hospitalization. This
typification work (indexically) singles out a certain aspect of an individual's
multifaceted presence in a particular context. This aspect is (documentarily)
interpreted as an "indicator" of the individual's membership in a more general
classification of persons (that is, the mentally ill). The diagnoser then (reflexively) "sees," in the labeled individual, a variety of attributes that typcially go
along with the "discovered" deviant membership. The seeing of these attributes
is taken to represent a seeing of who the individual really is (that is, a dangerous
or mentally ill person). The labeled individual is no longer just any individual. He
or she has been transformed into a certain type of person with a set of accompanying attributes.

The multifaceted presence of an individual at any one point in space and time suggests that he or she could hypothetically be categorized along an infinite set of idiosyncratic dimensions. Such multiple classification, however, would confound a labeler's own need to deal practically with the individual in a world which demands finite social responses. As such, the typification process routinely involves a search for pivotal categories by which to deal with the labeled other. I follow Lofland in suggesting that the attribution of deviance is one such pivotal category.[93]

In considering the typification or pivotal categorization of a patient as mentally ill, dangerous, in need of hospitalization, etc., I shall attend to how diagnosticians make interpretive use of such things as the setting of a patient's alleged deviance, a patient's nonaction personal effects or appearance, a patient's known or perceived activities, and the outcomes believed to be associated with a particular diagnostic label. Also considered will be the manner in which imputational specialists determine and use attributions of a patient's responsibility for his or her deviance, similarities or differences between a patient's values and theirs, and records of past typifications.[94]

The second stage of diagnostic work focuses on decisions to designate a patient publicly as this or that type of deviant. In this stage, the labeler is confronted with the choice to apply "publicly" the typical categorizations that have come to be known "privately" about a particular deviant. Will labeling agents call it as they see it or will such things as the consequences of public naming or the variant expectations of those who hear diagnostic pronouncements dissuade imputational specialists from applying a particular categorization? In what ways does the public designation of a deviant label depend on an imputational specialist's confidence in a given pivotal categorization? Moreover, how is a "sense of confidence" in typing and public designating achieved? In what ways is this confidence dependent on the number of available indicators suggesting a particular diagnostic label, on the credibility of indicators, on a perceived consistency between indicators, and on perceived agreement or consensus of other labelers? These are the questions associated with this second stage. They focus on the work done by diagnosticians to present reasonable accounts of the adequacy of particular labels and of the appropriateness of public designations.

The third stage in the production of diagnostic labels centers on the reworking or renegotiating of deviant types and designations given the resistance of others. The possible results of this renegotiation include the defense and/or cognitive elaboration of a particular label, the modification of a label, or the abandoning of a label. Involved in this process are ways that labelers typify the credibility and power of the patients, other labelers, or outside audiences who resist their attributions of deviance. Also involved is the degree to which the situated identity of labelers as imputational experts has become invested in particular typifications or designations. To be considered in examining this stage are various negotiated exchanges of deference, power, and "face" among labelers, their targets, and their audiences.

*To Accomplish a "Sense of Structure" by Naming
Patients as Types of Persons*

We are here defining the end-product of diagnostic work. The success of the attribution process is the accomplishment of a "sense of structure" concerning how, who, or what a patient really is. This success is paradoxically generated by the work of actors to sustain the experience of a "correspondence or matching theory" of their knowledge of patients. The names that become attached to a patient's condition come to be viewed not as products of the labeler but as "discoveries" about the labeled. Thus, it is assumed that "creating the reality of deviance" involves an interpretive transformation through which labelers typify their own work as "naming deviance as it really is." The strengths or merits of this assumption, of course, are dependent on its empirical demonstration in the analysis and display of our data.

*In Accordance with Their Own Perceived Interests*

The labeling process may be undertaken by imputational specialists in accordance with a variety of perceived interests. These interests may be conceptualized in terms of two general categories: perceived purposes-at-hand and situated identities. The purposes for doing diagnosing may include such diverse things as the need to cope with an unknown entity, an attempt to make some extra money, the intention of increasing professional competence or prestige, an effort either to save society or help patients, or even to get on the good side of one's diagnostic peers. By situated identity we refer to the work of actors who accomplish a particular sense or definition of self (for self or others) in the process of a particular course of action. For the Lima diagnosers such identities as "competent expert," "dedicated reformist," or "good guy who'll help out on the weekend" are all possible "identities" which may play a part in the type of work that diagnosticians actually do.

The relevance of perceived interests may vary across different work contexts.[95] Their importance, however, lies in their potential for becoming self-typified rationales for the interpretive work of psychiatric decision-making. This is true both for purpose-at-hand, typified as "I'm doing this or that in-order-to," and for situated identities, typified as "I'm doing this or that because I'm a certain kind of person." As such, these self-typified reasons for acting become additional "indexically relevant" features of the interpretive context in which diagnostic work is accomplished: thus, the "interests" of psychiatrist professionals, the relevance of their self-typified motives, and the identities of their interpretation of the task at hand.

It should be recognized that our phenomenological concern with the manner in which actors typify their interests and identities differs from social psychological research which posits that actors behave in certain ways because of certain motives or particular self-concepts. Our concern is chiefly with the interpretive work that diagnosticians do to typify their own purposes-at-hand and how the product of this self-typification functions as yet another codeterminant element of the context in which diagnostic work is being done. These issues bear a clear resemblance to symbolic interactionism's concern about knowledge of the self through making the self an object, considered through taking the perspective of others toward it.[96] They, likewise, resemble that tradition in attribution theory which suggests that "knowledge" of one's own motives is established in essentially the same way as "knowledge" of another's motives—by inferences from observed doings or behaviors.[97] Both of these traditions imply a process of dynamic assessment and fit conceptually with our prior definition of interpretive work.

The issue of self-typified motives and identities has only been marginally touched upon by ethnomethodology. Ethnomethodology has paid little, if any, attention to the problem of self-concept(ualizations). Our consideration of this issue, however, does not appear to contradict any elements of the ethnomethodological perspective. We are not suggesting that (labeling) actors work to establish self-typifications of their motives and situated identities and that the products of this work function as additional elements of the context in and through which (diagnostic) work is done. Hence, when we suggest that diagnostic work is done in accordance with actors' perceived interests, we are simply suggesting that an account of interpretive work must include an account of actors' own accounting practices in terms of relevant investments in particular purposes-at-hand and identities.

### And in Relation to the Resistance of Others

The area of resistance is also a topic which has been inadequately explored by ethnomethodology.[98] By resistance we refer to those experienced contextual and interactional constraints on the creativity of interpretive work. Ethnomethodology, of course, recognized that there is no pure documentary interpretation aside from the contextualizing process of indexical expression. Nonetheless, its emphasis on the lack of any social order aside from that constituted in the consciousness of the actor leads it to downplay resistance to the interpretive process. Such resistance is exercised by other actors against oneself. As Perinbanayagam points out in attempting to correct the "one-sidedness" of much ethnomethodological writing: "[The other actor] challenges the interpreter and asks him to explain himself, to extrapolate on his obscure and recalcitrant responses. And woe unto those who cannot and are also powerless—they may get carted off to an asylum."[99]

The limitations of ethnomethodology's inattention to the problem of resistance have also been recognized by recent sociological conflict theorists who argue that the unequal distribution of power constrains the interpretive process in a way not explicitly recognized by its adherents.[100] Perhaps this critique is best summarized by Dreitzel, who suggests that often "the breakdown of the norms of social action indicates a struggle over the rules of interpretation, a struggle which is, in its origin as well as outcome, dominated by factors alien to the interpretive creativity of the involved parties.[101]

Other "subjective perspectives" are not as vulnerable as ethnomethodology on the issue of resistance. As Maryl points out, symbolic interactionism overcomes this limitation by stressing that meaning is found only in the resistance or response of the other. The weakness of ethnomethodology is that it appears as a "sociology without society."[102] No wonder there is no systematic attention to resistances. According to Maryl, there is little systematic attention to anything outside of the actor's consciousness.

Although given little systematic attention, the issue of resistance does emerge as an implicit theme in a number of ethnomethodological studies. Certainly Garfinkel's students who were instructed to treat their parents as polite strangers began to experience the resistance of powerful others to their interpretive work. Many, we are told, had to stop their role-playing. The maintenance of their particular interpretations was being punished by the forceful resistance of others.[103] So, too, if one projects oneself into the position of "skid row" inhabitant, rather than of Bittner's observed policemen,[104] one would imagine it difficult to generate an acceptable interpretation of oneself as the overjoyous and affectionate lover of law officers. Imagine the indexical limits of the "skid row" alcoholic's interpretation of the reasonableness of holding hands and smooching with a policeman. It is an unlikely interpretation due to the negative outcomes that are indexically present for one who tries.

Ethnomethodology is not incapable of dealing with the issue of resistance. Obviously, this issue is implied in the very principle of indexicality. What is not spelled out clearly, however, is that the context of interpretation always presumes the existence of some others who, by virtue of their access to certain structural resources, offer various degrees of resistance to the work of interpretive reality construction. Some ethnomethodological studies have recognized this more than others. Indeed, Douglas's concern with the impact of power contexts on the production of social research,[105] Cicourel and Kituse's discussion of the constrained construction of official statistics,[106] and Daniel's study of psychiatric diagnoses[107] all suggest the ability of an ethnomethodological perspective to move in this direction. Yet, since the possibility of resistance is inherent in every social interaction, systematic attention to it reveals another important feature of the interpretive process—"the indexical interpretation of resistance." A systematic attention to this feature is a final theoretical commitment of the present analysis.

Our commitment to a consideration of the interpretative handling of resistances parallels that suggested by Prus.[108] He suggests that such matters as the degree of dissimilarity in offered types, the importance of the labeled target for the labeler, and the credibility of an alternative labeling source are all issues impacting on the receptiveness or defensiveness of labeling actors to information offered by other actors. Elsewhere, Prus discusses resistances buttressed by power, prestige, and knowledge differentials between labelers and between the labeled.[109] He argues that "[labeled] qualities are seen as highly problematic, reflecting both the interpretive frameworks of observers and the subsequent challenges of resisters contesting target attributions they consider inappropriate."[110]

In considering the diagnostic work of Lima patient review teams, it appears that resistance to labeling may stem from at least three sources: from the alternative interpretations of members within teams, from patients, and from the legal audience to whom diagnostic reports are submitted. Hence, a consideration of resistance and the role of perceived power, credibility, and knowledge differentials in defending, modifying, or abandoning certain diagnostic designations will be an integral feature of our analysis.

## Summary

We began this chapter by tracing the debate between labeling theory and the medical perspective on mental illness. It was argued that both parties to this debate distort the contribution of the societal reaction perspective on deviance by implicitly positing the necessary existance of a normative world prior to the scene of social interaction. On the other hand, the perspective of ethnomethodology was seen to have abandoned the normativity assumption in favor of an emphasis on the interpretive work of labeling agents in creating a "sense of normative rule violation." It was reasoned that this ethnomethodological perspective is more consistent with the theoretical intentions of the societal reaction perspective. As such, this perspective was selected as the theoretical basis for the present analysis of psychiatric decision-making.

We concluded this chapter with an outline of the various theoretical commitments which underlie our analysis of psychiatric decision-making. Before examining our substantive findings, however, I shall explore the practical methodological commitments which have guided the collection and analysis of our data. These methodological considerations provide the topic for our next chapter.

## Notes

1. John Kituse, "The 'New Conception of Deviance' and Its Critics," in Walter Gove, ed., *The Labelling of Deviance: Evaluating a Perspective* (New York: Halstead Press, 1975), p. 274.

2. Frank Tannenbaum, *Crime and the Community* (New York: McGraw-Hill Book Co., Inc., 1951).

3. George Herbert Mead, "The Psychology of Punitive Justice," *American Journal of Sociology* 23 (1918): 577-602.

4. Howard S. Becker, *Outsiders: Studies in the Sociology of Deviance* (New York: The Free Press, 1963).

5. Edwin M. Lemert, *Human Deviance, Social Problems and Social Control* (Englewood Cliffs, N.J.: Prentice Hall, 1972). This work expanded Lemert's earlier work within the societal reaction perspective, *Social Pathology* (New York: McGraw-Hill Book Co., Inc., 1951).

6. Howard Becker, p. 9.

7. Ibid.

8. Ibid., p. 10.

9. Thomas J. Scheff, *Being Mentally Ill: A Sociological Theory* (Chicago: Aldine Publishing Co., 1966).

10. Ibid., p. 93.

11. Thomas J. Scheff, "The Social Reaction to Deviance: Ascriptive Elements in the Psychiatric Screening of Mental Patients in a Midwestern State," *Social Problems* 11 (Spring 1964): 401-413. For an expanded consideration of this research see T. Scheff, *Being Mentally Ill.*

12. Various critiques of labeling theory were presented at the third Vanderbilt Sociology Conference (October 28-29, 1974). Papers presented at this symposium are collectively published in Walter R. Gove, ed., *The Labelling of Deviance: Evaluating a Perspective* (New York: Halstead Press, 1975).

13. Walter R. Gove, "Societal Reaction as an Explanation of Mental Illness: An Evaluation," *American Sociological Review* 35 (October 1970): 881.

14. This argument is made numerous times by advocates of the labeling position. See, for instance, Howard S. Becker, "Labelling Theory Reconsidered," in H.S. Becker, *Outsiders: Studies in the Sociology of Deviance* (New York: The Free Press, 1973), pp. 177-208; and Thomas J. Scheff, "The Social Reaction to Deviance."

15. Walter R. Gove, "Labelling and Mental Illness: A Critique," in W.R. Gove, ed., *The Labelling of Deviance: Evaluating a Perspective* (New York: Halstead Press, 1975), p. 35.

16. Walter R. Gove, "The Labelling Theory of Mental Illness: A Reply to Scheff," *American Sociological Review* 40 (April 1975): 242.

17. W.R. Gove, *The Labelling of Deviance*, p. 50.

18. Ibid., p. 51.

19. Ibid., p. 49.

20. Ibid., p. 51.

21. Marion Yarrow et al., "The Psychological Meaning of Mental Illness in the Family", *Journal of Social Issues*, Vol. 11, 4 (1955), pp. 12-24.

22. Gove in *The Labelling of Deviance*, cites support for his position in

56

such work as that of Harold Sampson, Sheldon Messinger, and Robert Towne, "The Mental Hospital and Marital Family Tree," *Social Problems* A (Fall 1961): 141-155; and Erving Goffman, *Relations in Public* (Garden City, N.J.: Doubleday, 1971), p. 357.

23. W.R. Gove, *The Labelling of Deviance*, p. 42.

24. Elliot Mishler and Nancy Wexler, "Decision Processes in Psychiatric Hospitalization," *American Sociological Review* 28 (August 1963): 576-587; and Weiner Mendel and Samuel Rapport, "Determinants of the Decision for Psychiatric Hospitalization," *Archives of General Psychiatry* 20 (March 1969): 321-328.

25. W.R. Gove, *The Labelling of Deviance*, p. 45.

26. Egon Bittner, "Police Discretion in Apprehending the Mentally Ill," *Social Problems* 14 (Winter 1967): 280.

27. Charles Tucker, "Demented Persons and Psychiatric Decisions" and "Societal Reactions and Mental Illness: An Examination of Police Behavior" (both unpublished mimeographs, 1972). The papers are described in W.R. Gove, *The Labelling of Deviance*, pp. 45-46. They apparently represent reports on a study of police and hospital records of persons brought for psychiatric treatment to a general hospital.

28. William Wilde, "Decision-Making in a Psychiatric Screening Agency," *Journal of Health and Social Behavior* 9 (September 1968): 215-221.

29. Dorothy Miller and Michael Schwartz, "County Lunacy Commission Hearings: Some Observations of Commitments to a State Mental Hospital," *Social Problems* 14, 1 (Summer 1966): 26-35.

30. W.R. Gove, *The Labelling of Deviance*, p. 46.

31. Muriel Hammer, "Influence of Small Social Networks or Factors on Mental Hospitalization," *Human Organization* 22 (Winter 1963-1964): 243-251.

32. W.R. Gove, *The Labelling of Deviance*, p. 52.

33. Bruce Dohrenwend and Barbara Dohrenwend, *Social Status and Psychological Disorder* (New York: John Wiley, 1969).

34. W.R. Gove, *The Labelling of Deviance*, pp. 52-53. See also Walter Gove and Patrick Howell, "Individual Resources and Mental Hospitalization: A Comparison and Evaluation of the Social Reaction and Psychiatric Perspectives," *American Sociological Review* 39 (February 1974): 86-100.

35. Jerome Myers and Bertram Roberts, *Family and Class Dynamics in Mental Illness* (New York: John Wiley, 1959). This trend is also said to be supported by the finding that well-educated ex-patients are generally the earliest hospital returnees. Shirley Angrist et al., *Women After Treatment: A Study of Former Mental Patients and Their Normal Neighbors* (New York: Appleton-Century-Crofts, 1968). The "lower tolerance" for deviance by middle-class families also reinforces this conclusion. Cf. Howard Freeman and Ozzie Simmons, "Social Class and Past Hospital Performance Levels," *American Sociological Review* 24 (June 1959): 345-351.

36. Jerome Myers and Lee Beam, *A Decade Later: A Follow-up of Social Class and Mental Illness* (New York: John Wiley, 1968).

37. W. Gove and P. Howell, "Individual Resources."

38. Joel Fisher, "Negroes and Whites and Rates of Mental Illness: Reconsideration of a Myth," *Psychiatry* 32 (November 1969): 428-446; Seymour Baxter, Nernard Chodorkoff, and Robert Underhil, "Psychiatric Emergencies: Dispositional Determinants and the Validity of the Decision to Admit," *American Journal of Psychiatry* 124 (May 1968): 100-104.

39. Walter Gove and Jeanette Tudor, "Adult Sex Roles and Mental Illness," *American Journal of Sociology* 28 (January 1973): 812-835.

40. Derek Phillips, "Rejection of the Mentally Ill: The Influence of Behavior and Sex," *American Sociological Review* 29 (October 1964): 679-687.

41. Ibid. For a summary of other recent findings in this same direction see Stuart Kirk, "The Impact of Labelling on Rejection of the Mentally Ill: An Experimental Study," *Journal of Health and Social Behavior* 15 (June 1974): 108-117.

42. Walter Gove and Terry Fain, "The Stigma of Mental Hospitalization: An Attempt to Evaluate Its Consequences," *Archives of General Psychiatry* 28 (April 1973): 494-500.

43. W. Gove, "Labelling Theory," p. 245.

44. Shirley Angrist et al., p. 176. Although not cited in this context by Gove, the work of Ann Davis, Simon Dinitz, and Benjamin Pasamonick, *Schizophrenics in the New Custodial Community* (Columbus, Ohio: The Ohio State University Press, 1974, appears to draw much the same conclusion.

45. W. Gove, "Labelling Theory," pp. 245, 247.

46. These rebuttals are contained in Thomas J. Scheff, "The Social Reaction to Deviance," and Thomas J. Scheff, "Reply to Chauncy and Gove," *American Sociological Review* 40, 2 (April 1975): 252-257.

47. Several recent studies clearly indicate that socioeconomic class is a major variable in facilitating attributions of some and impeding the application of other nosological designations. See particularly E. Gottheil, M. Kramer, and M.S. Huruich, "Intake Procedures and Psychiatric Decisions," *Comprehensive Psychiatry* 7 (1966): 207-215; J.F. McDermott et al., "Social Class and Mental Illness in Children: The Diagnosis of Organicity and Mental Retardation," *Journal of American Academy of Child Psychiatry* 6 (1967): 309-320; C.E. Shorer, "Mistakes in the Diagnosis of Schizophrenia," *American Journal of Psychiatry* 124 (1968): 1057-1062; R.I. Shader et al., "Raising Factors in Diagnosis and Disposition," *Comprehensive Psychiatry* 10 (1969): 81-89.

48. Thomas J. Scheff, "Reply," p. 253.

49. Ibid., p. 254.

50. Maurice Rappaport, "Selective Drug Utilization in the Management of Psychoses," paper read at the Western Psychological Association Meeting

(April 1973). Abstracted in *Psychology Today* 8 (November 1974): 39, 138. Scheff, "Reply," p. 256, also argues that a "hawthorne-like" effect may be operative in the use of tranquilizing drugs. This argument is not cited as a major rebuttal. The findings of other research, controlling for this effect through the use of placebo groups in an experimental design, appear to document the independent effect of drugs themselves. See B. Pasamanick, S. Dinitz, and F. Scarpitti, *Schizophrenics in the Community* (New York: Appleton-Century-Crofts, 1967).

51. The work of Bardach is cited as an example of the sociolegal impact of the labeling position in certain changes in mental health law. Cf. Eugene Bardach, *The Skill Factor in Politics: Repealing the Mental Health Commitment Laws in California* (Berkeley, Cal.: University of California Press, 1972).

52. Thomas J. Scheff, "Reply," p. 257.

53. Jack P. Gibbs, "Issues in Defining Deviant Behavior," in Robert A. Scott and Jack D. Douglas, eds., *Theoretical Perspectives on Deviance* (New York: Basic Books, 1972).

54. H. Becker, p. 20.

55. Thomas J. Scheff, *Being Mentally Ill,* pp. 31-32.

56. Ibid., p. 34.

57. Gibbs, pp. 56-64.

58. Actually our statement considerably reduces the complexity of the Gibbs formulation, which rejects the notion of unitary cultural norms while acknowledging degrees of normative violations and multiplicity of evaluative perspectives by which rule violations may be judged. For the present purposes, however, it is enough to say that Gibbs emphasizes evaluations of normative conduct as the basis for determining deviancy. See Gibbs, pp. 56-64.

59. Gibbs, pp. 48-49.

60. Ibid., p. 50.

61. This theme portraying the deviant as an underdog victimized by the social system has been criticized by "radical theorists" like Gouldner and Taylor, Walton and Young. Gouldner argues that this dimension by which labeling theory "romanticizes the victim" diverts serious attention from the problems of inequality and repression in the system as a whole. Taylor, Walton, and Young, on the other hand, argue that labeling theory tends to depoliticalize the meaning of a "deviant" actor's volitional struggle and resistance by converting him or her to the status of a meaningless product of victimization by others. Cf. Alvin Gouldner, "The Sociologist as Partisan: Sociology and the Welfare State," *American Sociological Review* 3 (May 1968): 103-116; Ian Taylor, Paul Walton, and Jack Young, *The New Criminology: For a Social Theory of Deviance* (London: Routledge and Kegan Paul, 1973).

62. John Kituse, p. 277.

63. Ibid. An excellent example of this "norms only upon reflection phenomenon" is found in Wallace's study of "dopers' " folk beliefs about

marijuana use. Consider the following report from Hugh Mehan and Houston Wood, *The Reality of Ethnomethodology* (New York: John Wiley and Sons, 1975), p. 163: "Wallace decided to validate his analysis . . . by asking dopers informally if smoking marijuana increased sensitivity. Wallace reports: 'On virtually all occasions the replies were positive, but the sense of most replies was one of realization, like "yea, that's a good way of talking about it." ' ". . . It was as if they had not thought of it before, but thought it was true once he mentioned it.' "

64. For further discussion of the correspondence or matching theory of knowledge see Mehan and Wood, pp. 182-190.

65. It should be remembered that Gibb's critique attends only to the labeling theory tradition within the societal reaction perspective. His observations do not address issues raised by the perspectives ethnomethodological tradition. This second tradition explicitly disavows the idea that "norms" or "rules" are "out there" independent of the actor. Hence, it also denies the utility of a correspondence theory of knowledge. The "substantive" elements of early labeling formulations (focusing on the processual creation of deviance) also appear to lean in this direction. A full exposition of this position is "distorted," however, by the "methodological" argument over "correctness." As Kituse argues, "The early statements by Lemert and Becker [and I suggest Scheff, as well] were importantly shaped by the conceptions that they opposed, so that they attempted to address old questions and issues even as they sought to establish and delineate a new perspective on deviance" p. 275). Also see John I. Kituse and Malcolm Spector, "Deviance and Social Problems: Some Parallel Issues," *Social Problems* 23 (Fall 1975).

66. Kituse, p. 277.

67. Ibid., p. 278.

68. Norman N. Gorgoff, "Simulation and Social Research: Incarceration and Subjective Meaning," a paper presented at the 1974 Meetings of the American Sociological Association, Montreal. It should be noted that Gorgoff's "inmates" were actually subjects simulating the role of inmates.

69. Jeff Coulter, p. 173.

70. Ibid., p. 175.

71. Ibid., p. 176.

72. J. Kituse, p. 278.

73. Cf. Kai T. Erikson, "Notes on the Sociology of Deviance," *Social Problems* 9 (1962): 307-314; John I. Kituse, "Societal Reaction to Deviant Behavior: Problems of Theory and Method," *Social Problems* 9 (1962): 247-256; Erick Goode, "Marijuana and the Politics of Reality," *Journal of Health and Social Behavior* 10 (1969).

74. Such terms as "cognitive sociology" or the "sociology of everyday life" have been recently offered as alternatives to the word ethnomethodology. The familiarity of the term ethnomethodology to students of deviance,

however, recommends its usage in the present context.

75. This definition reduces the wide range of complex issues that have fallen within the domain of ethnomethodology. It is believed consistent, however, with both Garfinkel's orginal usage and with Cicourel's elaboration of the topic in terms of the production of a sense of structure (surface rules) through the use of interpretive procedures (deep-seated rules). Cf. Harold Garfinkel, *Studies in Ethnomethodology* (Englewood Cliffs, N.J.: Prentice-Hall, Inc., 1967) and Aaron V. Cicourel, *Cognitive Sociology: Language and Meaning in Social Interaction* (New York: The Free Press, 1974).

76. H. Garfinkel, *Studies.*

77. Aaron V. Cicourel, "Basic and Normative Rules in the Negotiation of Status and Role," in H. Dreitzel, ed., *Recent Sociology No. 2* (New York: Macmillan, 1970), pp. 4-48; "The Acquisition of Social Structure: Toward a Developmental Sociology of Language and Meaning," in J. Douglas, ed., *Understanding Everyday Life: Toward a Reconstruction of Sociological Knowledge* (Chicago: Aldine, 1970), pp. 136-168.

78. A Cicourel, "Acquisition," and Peter K. Manning, "Talking and Becoming: A View of Organizational Socialization," in J. Douglas, ed., *Understanding Everyday Life* (Chicago: Aldine, 1970), pp. 239-256.

79. H. Garfinkel, p. 3.

80. Ibid., pp. 7-9.

81. H. Mehan and H. Wood, pp. 166-67.

82. The implications of "reflexivity" for the self-masking of social phenomenan is a major concern of Peter Berger and Thomas Luckmann's *The Social Construction of Reality* (New York: Doubleday, 1966). The authors describe this reification in terms of the three-phase process ot externalization-objectification-legitimation. A specific application of this perspective to the problem of deviance is found in H. Taylor Buckner, *Deviance, Reality and Change* (New York: Random House, 1971).

83. Melvin Pollner, "Sociological and Common-Sense Models of the Labeling Process," in Roy Turner, ed., *Ethnomethodology: Selected Readings* (Middlesex, England: Penguin Books, 1974), pp. 27-40.

84. The reader familiar with the phenomenological sociology of Schutz or the phenomenological analysis of Husserl, but not with the language of ethnomethodology, may wish to compare the closeness of the phenomenological notion of "appresentation" with the everyday strategy of "documentary interpretation." Cf. Alfred Schutz, *Collected Papers I: The Problem of Social Reality* (The Hague: Nijhoff, 1962), pp. 294-300. Those familiar with "attribution theory" in social psychology will also find similarities with the concerns of ethnomethodology. For example, Fritz Heider's explication of the workings of "naive psychology," in attributing a "causal structure" to another's behavior, is very similar to the method of documentary interpretation. Likewise, Heider's search for the invariant structures which underlie person perception parallels Cicourel's concern with "deep structures" and "the invariant proper-

ties" of interpretive rules." Cf. Fritz Heider, *The Psychology of Interpersonal Relations* (New York: Wiley, 1958).

85. Harold Garfinkel, "The Common Sense Knowledge of Social Structures: The Documentary Method of Interputation in Lay and Professional Fact Finding", in H. Garfinkel, p. 78.

86. H. Mehan and H. Wood, p. 75.

87. Ibid., p. 89. The openness of rules to the interpretive work of actors is also described by Garfinkel, who suggests that "events include as their essentially intended and sanctioned features an accompany 'fringe' of determinations that are open with respect to internal relationships, relationships to other events, and relationships to retrospective and prospective possibilities." Cf. H. Garfinkel p. 41.

88. W. Gove, "The Labeling Theory of Mental Illness, A Reply to Scheff," p. 245.

89. J. Kituse, p. 280.

90. John Lofland, *Deviance and Identity* (Englewood Cliffs, N.J.: Prentice-Hall, 1969), p. 139.

91. Ibid.

92. Our consideration of a multi-stage process model of diagnostic work is indebted to Prus's systematic analysis of the labeling process. Prus is working from the combined perspectives of symbolic interactionism and attribution theory. His conceptualization of the process of deviant attribution, except perhaps for a lack of explicit attention to the issue of "reflexivity," is very similar to that employed in the present analysis. Cf. Robert C. Prus, "Labelling Theory: A Reconceptualization and a Propositional Statement on Typing," *Sociological Focus* 8, 1 (January 1975): 79-96.

93. John Lofland, p. 124.

94. Most of the issues to be considered are detailed in propositional form by Prus, who introduces what might be construed as a "concatenated" model of deviance attribution. Cf. Prus, pp. 84-91.

95. In the broadest sense our use of the term "relevance" refers to the three types distinguished by Schutz: thematic, interpretational, and motivational relevance. The indexical constraints that any of these three types place on the interpretive work of diagnosticians is, of course, an important element of the experiential or phenomenological context in which this work occurs. Most specifically we are focusing on actors' work in typifying their own "in order to" motives in given contexts of social interaction. Cf. Alfred Schutz and Thomas Luckmann, *Structures of the Life World* (Evanston, Ill.: Northwestern University Press, 1973).

96. George H. Mead, *Mind, Self and Society* (Chicago: University of Chicago Press, 1932).

97. Daryl Bem, *Beliefs, Attitudes and Human Affairs* (Belmont, Cal.: Brooks/Cole, 1970).

98. The issue of resistances has also been explored by the author

elsewhere. Cf. Stephen J. Pfohl, "Social Role Analysis: The Ethnomethodological Critique," *Sociology and Social Research* 59, 3 (April 1975): 243-265.

99. R.S. Perinbanayagam, "The Definition of the Situation: An Analysis of the Ethnomethodological and Dramaturgical View," *Sociological Quarterly* 15 (August 1974): 539.

100. Ian Taylor, Paul Walton, and Jack Young, *The New Criminology: For a Social Theory of Deviance* (London: Routledge and Kegan Paul, 1973).

101. Hans Peter Dreitzel, *Recent Sociology No. 2: Patterns of Communicative Behavior* (New York: Macmillan, 1970), p. xviii.

102. William Maryl, "Ethnomethodology: Sociology Without Society," *Catalyst* 7 (Winter 1973): 15-28. Similar theoretical criticisms of ethnomethodology's relative inattention to power have also been raised in Bary Smart, *Sociology, Phenomenology and Marxian Analysis* (London: Routledge and Kegan Paul, 1976) and Anthony Giddens, *The New Rules of the Sociological Method: A Positive Critique of Interpretive Sociology* (New York: Basic Books, 1977).

103. Harold Garfinkel, "Studies of the Routine Grounds of Everyday Activities," in H. Garfinkel, pp. 47-49.

104. Egon Bittner, "Police Discretion."

105. Jack Douglas, *Understanding Everyday Life: Toward a Reconstruction of Sociological Knowledge* (Chicago: Aldine, 1970), p. 30.

106. Aaron V. Ciourel and John I. Kituse, "A Note on the Use of Official Statistics," *Social Problems* 11 (1963): 139-159.

107. Arlene Daniels, "Social Construction."

108. Robert C. Prus, "Labelling Theory."

109. Robert C. Prus, "Resisting Designations: An Extension of Attribution Theory into a Negotiated Contest," *Sociological Inquiry* 45, 1 (1975): 3-14.

110. Ibid., p. 11.

# 4

## Doing the Study: Methodological Considerations

*In order to capture the participants "in their own terms" one must learn their analytic ordering of the world, their categories for rendering explicable and coherent the flux of . . . reality. That, indeed, is the first principle of qualitative analysis.*

John Lofland, *Analyzing Social Setting*[1]

The work of evaluation team members, in constructing psychiatric understandings, definitions, and recommendations, provides the substantive focus for this book. The focus for the present chapter, however, is methodological. It is written so as to acquaint the reader with the methods by which we as researchers studied the methods by which psychiatric professionals arrived at assessments about patients.

### A Triangulated Field Study

Methodologically our work can best be described as a triangulation of field research strategies, each contributing a different vantage point from which to study the diagnostic process in the natural setting in which it occurs.[2] Our primary mechanism of data collection was the placement of seven researchers as observers during 135 of the approximately 700 patient reviews. These observers, situated as unobtrusively as possible, were able to witness social interaction occuring before, during, and after the psychiatric team members' interviewing of patients. The presence of these observers, of course, required the informed consent of both patients and clinicians. Observers contributed two types of data: their own observational notes and verbatim tape recordings of all that conversationally occurred during the selected patient reviews. Transcriptions from these recordings and excerpts from observers' notes constitute a major portion of the data analyzed and displayed in the substantive sections of this book.

As a supplement to observational and tape-recorded materials, in-depth interviews with the participating psychiatric professions were conducted shortly after the completion of the patient review project as a whole. During these interviews, review team members were questioned regarding their impressions, opinions, and reflections concerning both the patient reviews and the presence of the observer-researchers.

In addition to the observations, taped recordings, and team member interviews, several other sources of data were gathered in order best to understand the patient reviews within the socio-medical-legal context in which they were ordered and carried out. The further data sources included: (1) observations of two of the three cases in which patients appealed their original review recommendations to a representative of the overseeing federal court; (2) a review of the formal written recommendations that the assessment teams presented to the federal court; (3) interviews with the major legal actors involved in the generation and execution of the court order itself; (4) interviews with state mental health officials concerning their reactions to the court-ordered patient review process; (5) a review of selected patient records in order to familiarize ourselves with the historical and clinical materials that team members themselves used; (6) a collective interview with three designated patient leaders in order to gain some insight into the way that patients themselves viewed and/or prepared for the review process.

We are confident that our use of multiple data sources (triangulation) affords an understanding of the psychiatric assessment process that a single source of data by itself could not yield. The tape recordings offer a rich and reliable source for repetitively listening to and analyzing diagnostic conversations. On the other hand, observers were able to provide descriptions about a wide range of nonverbal interactional issues that would not find their way into the microphones of our audio recording equipment. Likewise, our interviews with the previously observed diagnosers allowed us access to the ways that these clinicians made sense (at least retrospectively) of what they did and why they did it. During the remainder of this chapter we shall examine some of the more practical or strategic problems encountered in the execution of this type of field research.

**Preparing to Enter the Field**

The seven observers selected for this project included three Ph.D.-level graduate students and four advanced (or recently graduated) undergraduate sociology majors. All had been exposed to the principles of field research in courses and class projects. Four had previous experience as observers in previous field research projects. Prior to entering the field each observer participated in approximately ten hours of specialized training exercises and meetings. In these sessions we considered the kinds of behaviors and interactions that would be the targets for our observations, the types of coding and note-taking procedures that would be most useful to our work in the field, and reviewed information concerning Lima State Hospital, the kinds of patients we would be seeing, and the social and legal basis for the court-ordered reviews.

In training sessions, researchers initially rehearsed observational skills by watching and comparing notes about video-taped group decision-making discussions. Subsequent training focused on observing the interactions of actors "role-playing" the interactional work of psychiatric review teams and patients. Of primary concern in these training sessions was sensitizing observers to such things as those interactional gestures which may indicate various phases of the decision-making process, those which suggest deference or dominance, and those which reflect the emotional states of participants and changes in such states. Observers were instructed that they would primarily be "nonparticipant" watchers of team members' interactions. They were requested to position themselves in the actual research setting as unobtrusively as possible. They were also instructed to provide detailed descriptions of the spatial positioning of members in relation to each other, of the physical appearance of all participants, and of all interactional incidents between team members and/or patients and the observer.

A commitment to "unstructured" descriptions entails by necessity a recognition of the interpretational work of the observers in particular contexts of nonrepeated social interaction. As such, it cannot be claimed that two observers would have seen an interactional sequence in "exactly the same way." Observers, unlike their taping equipment, are inherently interpreters, rather than recorders, of data. Their reports will always be informed by their own efforts to make sense out of what they see happening. In order they they might best approach reporting the situation in its own terms, it was decided that observers should describe what they saw in as much detail as possible. This procedure would not eliminate the interpretational or judgmental work of observers. It would, however, document the grounds for descriptive interpretation. For example, rather than reporting that a psychiatrist appeared to be dominant in a group discussion, observers were instructed to outline the kinds of gestures, things said, spaces occupied, and timings used to indicate to them that a psychiatrist was dominant. Instead of reporting that team members appeared to prejudge a patient's case before interviewing the individual, observers were asked to note what specific interactions, ploys, statements, expressions, or body movements provided the base for such an inference.

The commitment to unstructured but detailed observational description was supplemented by another "standardizing" strategy. It required observers to make reports on a number of similar issues for every patient review. This approach recognized both the situational uniqueness of each instance of interpretive work and the potentially transituational presentation of certain interactional problems about which we were concerned. Observers were thus asked to address eight questions for each session that they observed. (These questions, and several others added later in the project, are included in the following section on refining the field strategies.)

The questions for observers served to "focus observations." They were not intended to deflect attention from the natural sequencing and signification of events by members themselves. If, for instance, the physical use of records or body positioning was not seen as relevant to a particular scene of social interactions, observers could simply note this in their descriptions. These questions were, in other words, developed and formulated as guidelines, not constraints. They operated on the assumption that at least "somewhat common information" could be obtained on each of these issues for each patient review. They did not interfere with the notation of "somewhat unique information" on any other relevant issues for each review.

**Refining Our Field Strategies**

During the course of its observational work the research team met once a week on Wednesday nights to compare notes, discuss problems, arrange schedules, and suggest modifications in the data collection and recording process. These weekly meetings provided a wealth of informal (if often anecdotal) data and also provided the basis for questions that would later be asked during the subsequent team member interviews. Comments made during these meetings also led to a modification of our system of observer note-taking. Observers, who occasionally saw as many as ten patient review sessions in a given day, were finding it exceedingly difficult to produce detailed and accurate notes which also addressed each of the previously mentioned observer questions for each review session watched. Some observers (who had other jobs and responsibilities) were finding it necessary to return to the field six days after completing their last observations (since the reviews took place largely on consecutive weekends) without having completed their notes from the session before.

Falling behind in note completion presented more than merely a practical pressure problem. We soon became concerned about the impact of current observations on the writings of previous observational accounts. As such, we shifted our observational notation system to a debriefing procedure involving the in-depth interviewing of observers about what they saw shortly after they saw it. These debriefing interviews by researchers with researchers usually lasted about two hours. They manifested several distinct advantages over the original procedure for elaborating observer notes. A first advantage of this method was that it guaranteed that each observer addressed the basic substantive concerns of the project for each team observed. The debriefing questionnaire was devised so as to focus attention on thirteen different areas of concern. These included such general categories as descriptions of preinterview, interview, and postinterview behavior, status-power relationships, and participant attentiveness. Also included were questions regarding a team's attitude toward a patient, a team's attitude toward the patient review process, a team's use of patient records, and a physical description of the appearance of a patient (his or her physical condition, dress, and demeanor). Observers were additionally asked about their own reaction to a patient, their affect toward a particular team, and their perceptions about their own impact on the interactional setting, and they were given the opportunity to make any additional observations of any sort.

Other advantages of the debriefing method were that it allowed the debriefing interviewers to probe for detailed documentation of the basis for observer influences; it permitted researchers to write less (and watch more) during actual observation sessions; it reminded observers, who carried debriefing questionnaires with them, to pay focused attention to the issues about which they would later be questioned; and it provided the research coordinator (who would later have to write up the "findings" for the whole project) a more extensive firsthand contact with observers' own reports of their experiences. This technique proved to be a more helpful vehicle for being in touch with what other observers saw happening and for ensuring that common issues were addressed in all observations. In addition, it provided a neatly structured format for storing the observational data. Coded extractions from the debriefing through debriefing questionnaire.

The Wednesday-night researcher meetings also provided an opportunity for researchers collectively to suggest solutions for "jams" or troublesome situations that were encountered in their roles as observers. In this sense, the meetings were didactic. They represented a forum for the ongoing instruction and training of the researchers in how to handle themselves in the field. A review of the tape recordings of these meetings (somewhat of an electronic log recording the "natural history" of this study) suggests four "trouble-solution" themes that emerged and reemerged in conversations among researchers. These "jams" and their suggested solutions are outlined below. It should be recognized, however, that our simple statement of such themes (included to give the reader a "feel" for what we encountered as investigators) is but an abstract reduction of many, many hours of shared experience, struggles, and reformulations.

*Theme One: How Best to Develop Rapport While Simultaneously Maintaining a Distance from Personal Involvement*

Researchers were instructed to take the role of the nonparticipant observer. They were asked to observe team decision-makers without becoming coproducers in their psychiatric decisions. It was believed that a good working relationship or sense of professional rapport with team members was needed in order to accomplish one's role as an unobtrusive observer. It was similarly believed that too much personal rapport could lead to a situation in which observers would begin to exercise a significant impact in the formulation of decisions. Thus observers were asked to play a politely professional role in which they appeared busy with their own work and disinterested in engaging team members in person-to-person relationships. They were asked to be friendly, but not friends; honest, but not open to further involvement; courteous, but not self-revelatory or personally inquiring.

*Theme Two: How to Be Polite But Substantively Non-responsive to Participant Requests for Observer Information*

This theme runs hand in hand with the "polite distance from personal involvement" theme. It emerged in discussions concerning how to handle requests for input by team members. It was suggested that observers should respond by politely stressing that for them to answer such questions would bias or endanger the objectivity of their research.

*Theme Three: How Best to Explain the Research*

Despite the fact that there were no hidden hypotheses in our research, some team members asked researchers what it was that they were "really" looking for. Researchers were instructed to rattle off prepared answers in sociological jargon, referring to such matters as "a systematic exploration of the social interaction dynamics of collective decision, etc." This "sociological jargon" explanation was perceived as both honest and efficient. A study of interactional work of diagnosticians was truly the focus of our investigation. The observers were neither "checking up" on the teams nor just performing an assigned student exercise. They needed to come across as professional yet not threatening.

*Theme Four: How Best to Prevent Observer Note-Taking from Interfering in Participant Decision-Making*

In the research meetings it was frequently reported that in the early weeks of the project, members of certain review teams repeatedly tried to see what it was that the observers were jotting down in their notes. In discussing this matter with other observers, it was noted that a certain few team members appeared more concerned with this issue than did others. Nonetheless, observers were instructed to position themselves in such a way that team members would be less tempted and less able to attempt to "read over an observer's shoulder." Observers were also asked to minimize eye contact with participants who appeared particularly interested in what they were about and to use shorthand notations to keep detailed writing to a minimum. Rather than write everything out in the presence of participants, observers were reminded to make concise notes which they could enflesh after leaving the scene of observation.

Modifying our note-taking system and dealing with troublesome inter-actional jams were issues that arose in the course of being in the field. A third issue generated, as it were, by the field concerned the manner in which we arranged our observations.

At the outset of the project it was hoped that during the course of field-work each observer would have the opportunity to observe each of the twelve review teams. We also hoped to accumulate a minimum of ten taped observations per team. It was believed that the achievement of these numerical idealizations would maximize the comparability of our sample between observers and between teams.

Upon entering the field we soon recognized a number of practical contingencies which limited our numerical idealizations. Although most review teams worked on each Saturday and Sunday, some worked one day and not the other, while a few others worked only one weekday each week. This staggered scheduling, combined with the fact that some teams did not really show up at the times for which they were scheduled, conflicted with the availability of certain observers at certain times. Moreover, the review teams worked at an unanticipatedly rapid pace and actually finished their evaluation in seven rather than the mandated sixteen weeks. Furthermore, as might be expected, some review teams worked faster (or diagnosed more patients) than others. These several unexpected contingencies shortened the term of our field observations and decreased the proportionality of the number of diagnoses we saw per team (given our unit for a day's observations as "accompanying a team during its entire day's work").

In spite of the contingencies described above, only one observer had to observe the same team twice (once early and once late in the project) and only one team of the twelve teams was never observed (a team working only on one weekday). Nonetheless, because of the rapid work of certain teams, we had (in less than half the projected time) observed and recorded more review sessions than originally anticipated. As stated previously, we had hoped to observe ten sessions for each of twelve teams. This would have given us a total of 120 observed reviews. As it turned out, we recorded data on 135 patient reviews. The distribution of reviews and observers among teams was, however, less balanced than our idealized projections. While ten represented the median number of reviews, the distribution ranged from four to twenty-two. The distribution of observers per team ranged from one to five. The median number of observers was three. These figures are presented in the following table. Teams are coded anonymously according to randomized alphabetization.

The comparability of observations between observers is obviously reduced by our final contingency-determined sampling of patient reviews. Yet, a

**Table 4-1**
**Distribution of Observations and Observers per Review Team**

| Team | Number of Reviews Observed | Number of Observers |
|---|---|---|
| A | 6 | 1 |
| B | 21 | 4 |
| C | 19 | 4 |
| D | 4 | 1 |
| E | (not observed in operation) | – |
| F | 4 | 1 |
| G | 14 | 4 |
| H | 9 | 2 |
| I | 10 | 2 |
| J | 18 | 4 |
| K | 5 | 3 |
| L | 25 | 5 |
| Totals | 135 | 30 |

qualitative analysis of a team's approach, style, assumptions, and negotiated interactions is not necessarily eliminated by the small numbers (that is, $N=4$) in a few of the observation cells. Indeed, most of the small numbered cells represent an entire day's diagnostic and decision-making work. Although it would obviously have been advantageous to contrast this one day's work with decision-making work done on other days, our analysis of a single sequence of interactions still yields considerable information on the kinds of interpretive strategies employed by a particular team. On the other hand, the six teams for which we have three or more separate observational segments provide us with data by which to assess the developmental history of certain diagnostic strategies. Hence, while the sampling is less balanced than originally anticipated, I feel reasonably confident that a consideration of the 135 separate cases provides a rich base of data for an analysis of the process of patient review.

### The Impact of Observers on Members' Work

Observers did not feel that they generally influenced or systematically biased the direction of patient reviews. This is not to say that they believed that their presence went unnoticed. Yet, the most consistent observation by all observers was that, following an initial period of mutual orientation, most teams and team members routinely accommodated the field researchers and showed little interest in or concern with their presence as observers. This observation is illustrated in the following observer comment.

Excerpt 3-1. From Observer Notes

Although the team members often at first seemed somewhat uncertain about my presence (which is understandable), in every case these people were friendly—and in many cases they were very considerate. In no case did members seem concerned about my competence. In any event, I did not pick up any cues indicating such a concern.

Nonetheless, my belief that observers did not systematically bias the general process of patient reviews is borne out by two other sources of data: the responses of team members during postreview work interviews and an analysis of tape-recorded observer-involved interactions. Each of these data sources will be examined in turn.

*Review Team Members' Assessments of Observers' Presence*

Near the end of the team member interviews (discussed in the following section) the psychiatric professionals were asked the following question. "As a final question—we'd like to know whether you felt the presence of research observers and tape recorders affected the way you performed your patient reviews. If so—in what ways?" The responses to this question fell into four categories. The first category contains responses to the effect that the presence of observers had *no impact* on members' work as psychiatric decision-makers. The second involved responses in which members believed observers has *some impact*, but that this impact had *no serious* effect on the style or direction of their work. A third category concerned responses in which members stated that observers had a *definite impact* in the direction of making the patient reviews *more formalized* or more serious. A fourth category included responses indicating that observers had a *definite impact* in *distracting* members from their work at hand. The following table summarizes the breakdown of members' responses to this question by their disciplinary status (that is, psychiatrist, psychologist, or social worker).

The responses recorded in table 4-2 support the field researchers' own assessment that their presence introduced little in the way of systematic impact or bias. Twenty-four of thirty-five respondents indicated that the presence of observers had no impact at all. Only three respondents stated that observers had a definite impact on the review proceedings. As it turned out, this small number coincided with the few concerned or critical individuals singled out in the researchers' own observations.

The following excerpt from an interview with a participating psychiatrist typifies the reaction of most review team members to the presence of research

**Table 4-2**
**Team Members' Assessment of Impact of Research Observer**

|  | Psychiatrist | Psychologist | Social Worker | Combined Decision Makers |
|---|---|---|---|---|
| No impact | 7 | 6 | 11 | 24 |
| Some impact/ not serious | 1 | 5 | 2 | 8 |
| Definite impact/ more formal | 1 | 0 | 0 | 1 |
| Definite impact/ distraction | 1 | 1 | 0 | 2 |
| No experience with observer, no response | 1 | 0 | 0 | 1 |
| Totals | $N$=11 | $N$=12 | $N$=13 | $N$=36 |

team members. Actually, several respondents, stating that their teams "would have done nothing differently," suggested that they were quite used to being observed and taped by student interns in their everyday work. Several others indicated only that they were disappointed that their teams "did not have observers more frequently."

Excerpt 3-2 From Psychiatrist Interview

It [their presence] didn't seem to bother anybody. It didn't bother the patient. . . . They were not obtrusive. They sat back and did their thing. I asked them if they would like to introduce themselves or if they wanted us to introduce them, and most of them said, "Well you just go ahead and introduce us," whoever's leading off . . . . They were nice to work with.

The general sense of six of the eight clinicians who noted that observers had some but no serious impact was that their own behaviors may have been a bit more formal and that they may have spent a bit more time with patients than may have been the case otherwise. The other two respondents in the "some impact/not serious" category believed that in a small number of cases the presence of a female observer may have distracted or affected the behavior of male patients. Yet both of these individuals later added that "most of the patients seemed to talk freely in the presence of an observer," and "for the most part it [the presence of observers] didn't seem to interfere."

Excerpt 3-3. From Psychologist Interview

Uh, the only influence it had, at least for me, was that in our discussions, you know, I tend to joke around a bit or kid a little bit. I think I was a little bit inhibited about that ... at least for a while. Later in the day. The observer that we had ... was really quite good, in terms of [that] we were comfortable with her, and she was comfortable with us and the patients were comfortable with her.

Of the three clinicians who indicated that observers had a "definite impact," one psychiatrist simply believed that "the interview probably went much more seriously," while another psychiatrist and a psychologist believed that they were distracted by not really knowing what the observer was looking for. It is significant to note that the "definite impact" beliefs of these singular respondents were not shared by their colleagues. In each case, members' coworkers indicated that observers had little or no impact.

### Observer-Involved Interactions

Other than when they were introduced for the purpose of explaining the research project and requesting a patient's informed consent to be observed, observer-focused interactions were rare occurrences during the patient reviews. Yet in analyzing tapes and transcripts two types of observer involvements were noted in a small number of the review sessions. The first of these concerns the use of observers (or patients' reactions to observers) as indicators of a patient's particular psychiatric reality. The most frequent examples of this have a clear "sexual undertone." Psychiatric team members are able to see in a patient's reaction to observers clear elements of a patient's heterosexual or homosexual urges. Concrete instances of this type of use of observers as indexes of a patient's mental status are discussed in subsequent sections of this monograph. One interesting use of an observer-involved interaction is worth noting at this point, however. It focuses on several patients' refusal to sign the observer consent form. This refusal had a clear impact on one team member. The nature of this impact is described below.

Excerpt 3-4 From Social Worker Interview

If you recall the first couple of patients didn't want to be taped. I respect that. That's OK. As a matter of fact, it may even have influenced me slightly. You know, perceiving the patient as being more related to reality. 'Cuz he didn't know you, he didn't know how you were going to use it, he didn't know whether he could trust you.

A second involvement concerned the use of observers as a "confirmation of a team member's thesis." This strategy was less frequent. It is

illustrated by the case of a team member who, in presenting a lengthy monologue on the social-cultural roots of a particular patient's problem, turned to the
observer and remarked, "I'm sure that you as a sociologist would, of course,
understand and agree with what I'm trying to explain." While the observer did
little more than respond with a nod of the head, the team member had accomplished a type of "cognitive coalition." The observer was here used as a supportive resource for a particular line of psychiatric theorizing.

The sporadic occurrences of "observer as indicator" and "observer as documentation" involvements do not suggest any real systematic distraction of the
review process by virtue of our observational presences. Together with the
previous analysis of feedback from both the observers and the observed, this
data leads to the conclusion that our observations did little to alter significantly
the phenomenon which we wished to watch. If anything, our presence made
the process (at least for some members) more formal and more rigorous. The
reader may wish to keep this in mind in considering the excerpted materials
that are to follow.

## Interviewing Team Members

Our approach to interviewing as conversational interaction was highly influenced
by Cicourel's discussion of this sociological practice in *Method and Measurement
in Sociology*.[3] We were convinced that together the questioner and respondent
structured a particular definition of social reality. We were, of course, interested
in allowing respondents to maximumly structure answers on and in their own
terms. We realized, however, that this idealized state of affairs could only be
partially approximated. Hence, we attempted to keep some natural history of
interview interactions in order to assess the manner in which interviewers influenced the flow of events and production of answers.

The use of tape recorders freed us from having to note the substantive
nature of respondents' answers. Interviewers were thus able to jot down interactional notations during the course of actual interviews. This practice was
additionally facilitated by the fact that approximately two-thirds of our interviews were jointly conducted by two members of the research team. They
allowed one member to conduct most of the questioning, while providing the
other with the opportunity to observe the overall flow of the interview and to
initiate substantive probes into various topics. Interview notes provided us with
a sense of how respondents reacted to certain questions in the course of an
interview. They also described the general interactional or interpersonal style of
a respondent and pointed out "slips" in our interviewing techniques or language.
These notes provided us with a basis for "indexing" the context of particular
responses and for reformulating our subsequent interview strategies.

In general a review of our notes on the social interactional character of our interviews led us to conclude that we were relatively successful in getting respondents to reconstruct verbally their own impressions of the patient review process. The confidence was strengthened by most interview notes, which reported a high degree of cooperation between psychiatric professionals and the sociological interviewers. This confidence in no way ignored the fact that all interviews were also social interactions. Our own work in approaching and questioning respondents undoubtedly represented the occasion for their various formulations. Being aware of this fact, we attempted to structure our interviewing so as to maximize the opportunity for respondents to speak for themselves about their own concerns and in their own terms. A "natural history" of our interview notes, discussions, and the taped interviews themselves, reveals five themes by which we structured our work as interviewers. A brief examination of these five themes should provide the reader with a sense of how we provided a social structure for the interviews themselves. This examination should further explicate the grounds for our confidence that respondents' answer to our questions were relatively representative of their own reconstructions about the diagnostic work they had performed.

## 1. Working on Respondents' "Home Grounds"

Our interviews were conducted in respondents' own offices or homes.[4] In arranging for interviews, we explained that we wished to talk with the respondents as resource persons who could provide us with additional understanding of the process of patient review. Our work, in other words, was geared toward achieving a situation in which respondents felt that they were operating on their own "home grounds."

It was our assumption that respondents' sense of being on their own home grounds would encourage them to be more "proactive" in reconstructing their patient review experiences. Surrounded by the spatial and social symbols of their own professional lives, it was hypothesized that respondents would feel more in control and be less "reactive" to the cues of interviewers concerning how to answer particular questions.

Going to the respondents also allowed us to maximize our number of interviews. We were able to conduct interviews with thirty-five of a target population of thirty-nine professionals. Two other respondents, while not availing themselves to an actual interview, completed a mailed questionnaire. This questionnaire contained all the questions that other respondents were asked in face-to-face interviewing. Thus, we were able to obtain interview or questionnaire data from thirty-seven of thirty-nine potential respondents.

The success of casting respondents into the role of resident expert is suggested by interviewers' observations concerning the manner in which respondents managed their physical and social environments. Most respondents were practicing clinicians. Their offices were typically arranged so as to differentiate between clinician or teacher spaces and client or learner spaces. We were guests in their offices and presented ourselves as coming to learn. We had to manage carefully our interactional work to ensure that respondents knew they had this sense of control and that we saw them in a resource person or teacher role. We sat where they guided us to sit. We attempted to manage our identities as "professional learners" who had come to hear "professional teachers."

The didactic answers that most respondents initiated allowed us to believe that respondents generally saw themselves in this teacher role. A somewhat humorous bit of anecdotal evidence provides additional support for this belief. In four instances the psychiatric professionals acutally attempted to bill the Division of Mental Health for the time they spent assisting us. For one psychiatrist, whose interview extended into a second hour of his day, a bill "for professional services rendered" totaled $100. We felt that we had profited as sociologists from the interview. The bill, however, led us to wonder later what type of help this individual believed that he actually had given us or which type he felt we needed most.

## 2. Working to Show Undifferentiated Interest

According to Hyman, interviews are inherently enfleshed with situated negotiations for definitions of what to do, say, and think which have not been previously anticipated, rehearsed, and standardized.[5] Our interviews were no exception. As explained above, our verbatim recordings and interview interaction notes simply provided a means for assessing the impact of negotiated social interaction. Our "general view" of interviewing, however, singled out two specific areas of social interaction for which we tried to approximate similar interviewer approaches or styles. The first of these concerned the issue of what to do about showing evaluative responses to respondent answers. The "neutral" or "cold-faced" approach to interviewer objectivity appeared to be highly problematic for our purposes. On one hand, it seemed that some show of interest would be necessary to maintain a conversational sense of interaction in which respondents would feel free to reconstruct their experiences in their own terms. On the other hand, it seemed likely that respondents would commonsensically attribute some evaluative tone to even the most "neutral" of intended interest gestures. Believing that respondents search for evaluation cues regardless of an interviewer's overt behavior, we decided to attempt to provide interest cues (smiles, nods, statements of interest) for all lines of a respondent's formulation. We attempted, in other words, to provide an undifferentiated positive response for all categories of respondent answers, rather than trying to act uniformly disinterested.

## 3. Working to Question and Probe "Innocently"

A second element of interview interactions with which we were particularly concerned focused on respondent efforts to attribute or typify our motives for asking certain questions or carrying out certain probes. Our "real" motives, as best as we could typify them, were simply to gain understanding of the perspectives employed by team members. As such, we tried to preface our various questions with lead-in descriptions of the reasons for asking them. For instance, in asking about leadership, we stated: "Leaders are often said to emerge in small groups of people interacting over a period of time. Would you say that a leader developed in your review team?" In asking about tension and conflict, we suggested: "Tension and conflict are also part of the process of most group interaction. Can you describe any point in the patient reviews in which members of your team were somewhat tense or in conflict with each other?"

In introducing certain probes at points in the interview we also ran the risk of raising respondent suspicion that we had some "hidden agenda." Review of the interview tapes reveals that interviewers frequently used what came to be referred to as "the Columbo approach" to probing "innocently." This technique was named after the television detective of the same name. It employed the reasoning that, since we're only sociologists (and not psychiatric professionals), we might not understand this or that "psychiatric topic." Hence, more information was requested without necessarily arousing respondents' suspicions that we didn't trust, honor, accept or think much of an original answer. The main thrust of this strategy was to get "innocently" an elaboration of an answer without putting a respondent on guard about revealing too much. It ordinarily resulted in more information without loss of rapport.

## 4. Working to Structure Reconstructing

The first three interview work themes were geared toward maximizing respondents' formulations in their own terms. The fourth concerns our development of an open-ended set of sixteen general topics of inquiry in order to provide some structured comparability among respondents' reconstructions. The questions within each topic were derived from concerns enumerated by observers during the course of the preceding field observations. They focused on the manner in which team members became initially involved in the review process, on a team's mode of organizational operation, on a member's assessment of his or her own input into team decisions, and on a team's leadership, conflict, and tension. Members were also asked to compare Lima patients with others and with clients they see in their everyday practices, to describe differences between the type and setting of the work they did at Lima and diagnostic work done elsewhere, to evaluate the helpfulness of the court order, and to describe in detail the specific strategies they employed to evaluate and classify various types of patients.

Members were also questioned as to any problems that their review teams may have encountered. They were asked to describe examples of easy and difficult cases, to reflect on their emotional reactions to patients, and to describe their own professional orientation and training. Final questions to respondents asked them to assess their confidence in their final decisions, their knowledge of other teams' work, the impact of medication on a patient's self-presentation, their knowledge of literature on the topic of diagnostic and predictive validity, and their impressions of the impact of observers on their work. The sequence of questions began with a general orientation inquiry and ended with an opportunity for respondents to make any additional comments that they so desired.

### 5. Working to Contain Feelings of Alienation

Interviewers sometimes identified with or agreed with the perspectives of some team members. They sometimes were dismayed by and disagreed with the perspectives of others. The problem with this was that our attempts at providing undifferentiated positive responses left us no vehicle for venting our disagreement. Occasionally interviewers, who had developed a certain compassion for Lima patients, were personally angered by what they perceived to be the cold or professionally mechanical responses of certain respondents. The following excerpt from an interviewer's notes illustrates one such experience:

Excerpt 3-5. From Notes on Interview with a Psychiatrist

I tried to assume the "Columbo" role by prefacing my questioning with the disclaimer that since I was only a sociologist I might not have a full clinical appreciation of the situation. I then repeated his explanation that it was in the very nature of a sociopath to try to manipulate a favorable presentation of self. He said that I was correct in my understanding. I then suggested that it must be difficult to decide on whether an individual is a sociopath in context of an interview. What if an individual expressed the belief that he or she had really changed or adjusted for the better? How would the clinician be able to decide if it was just the manipulations of sociopathy showing itself or whether the person was giving an honest answer and really had changed? I tried to phrase my questions to show sympathy with the difficult task of the clinician.

He responded by shaking his head and saying something like: "Well there's no problem there. They do try to manipulate you because they're sociopaths. You just have to see it." I thought initially that he had not understood my question and tried to rephrase my original inquiry. He sort of snickered and then replied to the effect that: "Well, see, they do try to manipulate you. They're sociopaths. That's why they're there. You just have to see the way they try to manipulate you." He concluded by saying that he really resented people who try to manipulate him and stated that he didn't like working on those "sociopath wards."

I couldn't believe it. He saw no inconsistencies, no circularities in his logic. I felt like laughing or screaming but instead smiled and heard myself say (very Rogerianly): "OK, I think I understand what you mean. Because they were there you know that they were sociopaths. So. What you had to do was look for the signs of manipulation." He agreed in a confident, matter-of-fact kind of way. I was furious "inside" but giving a nod of my head in feigned interest on the "outside." I felt horribly alienated and was glad that the interview was almost over so that I could share my feelings with the other interviewer.

Experiences such as that described above occurred in the course of a number of team member interviews. These experiences became typified and dealt with in terms of what we believed was the inherent alienation involved in this kind of fieldwork. We didn't feel comfortable. We knew that in terms of our total personhoods, we were playing a false role consciously, being and feeling phony. Our rationalization was that without such an experience we could not have obtained as clear a sense of the respondent's own perspective. At the same time we know we were confronting an existential dilemma at the heart of sociological research itself and could only support each other in the hope that we would ultimately use the knowledge we obtained toward the ends of de-alienating our daily lives and the world in which we live.

*The Analysis That Follows*

In the preceding pages we have tried to acquaint the reader with how it was that we obtained the data upon which we reported. In the subsequent analysis I shall endeavor to provide as much "firsthand" access to this data as possible. I believe firmly that verbatim references to and displays of observed materials strengthen our claim of being true to the perspectives and practices of the clinicians we observed. The verbatim transcripts, presented in excerpted form, are analyzed as typical instances of a complex process we observed over and again. This data is occasionally fragmented, as in the case of a technical recording error, an inaudible utterance, or an instance where a particular tape expired and had to be changed. In general, however, the excerpted transcripts represent relatively complete, verbatim reports of what was said by psychiatric decision-makers during or after and about the diagnostic process.

The editorial form in which transcribed excerpts are presented (punctuation and sentence structure, etc.) is designed so as to preserve, as much as possible, the original constructions and emphases of the observed participants. However, we have chosen not to elaborate our editing in the more technical fashion of analysts whose central substantive concern is with the social production of conversation as a phenomenon in its own right.[6] While consistent editing for things such as inflection, speaker overlap, and timing of pauses may facilitate a more detailed examination of the structure of talk itself, it may also complicate transcripts in such a fashion as to distract from the central substantive theme of our own work—the interactional production of particular versions of psychiatric reality. With this in mind we have chosen to simplify this presentation of transcribed data, substituting for detailed, line-by-line technical editing a series of parenthetical editorial comments informing the reader of relevant, contextual features that are not evidenced in the words themselves.

It is our hope that, in simultaneously reviewing the data presented, along with our interpretations of it, the reader will be able to decide on the "plausible" or "objective" character of our own interpretive accounts. This should strengthen our claims to have found out certain things about the social dynamics of the diagnostic process. At the same time, the presentation of verbatim materials permits the reader to join with us in the analytic process and offer an alternative interpretation should one appear more plausible. In any event, the following chapters are offered as an experience for learning about the social interactional process that is a part of diagnostic psychiatric work.

### Notes

1. John Lofland, *Analyzing Social Settings* (Belmont, Cal.: Wadsworth Publishing Co., 1971), p. 7.
2. Our conception of triangulation as a research strategy is derived from Norman K. Denzin, *The Research Act in Sociology* (London: Butterworths, 1970), pp. 297-313.
3. Aaron V. Cicourel, *Method and Measurement in Sociology* (New York: The Free Press, 1964), pp. 102-103.
4. A notable exception to this was one interview conducted with a respondent at a cafeteria location rather than a professional office. It is interesting to mention that in this instance interviewers observed an "untypical" uneasiness and a somewhat defensive attitude on the part of the respondent.
5. Herbert Hyman et al., *Interviewing in Social Research* (Chicago: University of Chicago Press, 1954), p. 57.
6. For a guide to the type of technical editing symbols used in much "conversational analysis" see Emmanuel A. Schegloff "Notes on a Conversational Practice: Formulating Place," in David Sudnow, ed., *Studies in Social Interaction* (New York: The Free Press, 1972), pp. 75-119.

**Part III
Substantive Findings**

# 5

## Introducing the Actors: Psychiatric Professionals and Their Patients

*The most distinctive part of the order was [that] the Court required people at Lima to be evaluated against some sort of valid standard for commitment to see if all patients really belong there.*

> Excerpt from statement of Justice Department attorney participating as an "amicus curiae" in case of *Davis* v. *Watkins*[1]

The court order to reevaluate each patient confined within the maximum-security setting of Lima State Hospital was part of a larger process of right-to-treatment litigation challenging the standards and practices of treatment for Ohio's "criminally insane." Although the idea of reviewing all patients actually arose in the course of casual conversations among attorneys, it was soon viewed by all parties (and agreed to in a consent decree) as an important first stage in securing patients' civil rights.[2] Lawyers representing the patient-plaintiffs expressed confidence that these reviews were carried out by "some of the leading experts in the state of Ohio." It was believed that these reviews would (as a first step in a reform process) remove those patients who really didn't belong in maximum security in the first place. According to one attorney, this inter-disciplinary review process "is important because it brings mental health professionals who have an unbiased, fresh view towards the patient into the institution for the first time."[3]

Clearly the legal actors who developed the case on behalf of Lima State's approximately 700 patients viewed the patient review process with both confidence and reformist expectations. In this chapter I shall provide background information on the two major categories of actors involved in this process: psychiatric professionals and the patients they diagnosed. I am, in a sense, introducing the actors and hence setting the stage for the subsequent analysis of their interactions.

### The Psychiatric Team Members

Thirty-seven clinicians were selected to participate in the patient review process. This included eleven psychiatrists, thirteen psychologists, and thirteen psychiatric social workers. All were chosen in accord with the court's rather stringent

83

guidelines for a "qualified mental health professional."[4] These guidelines guaranteed that all psychiatrists would be licensed and board certified, that all clinical psychologists would be accredited Ph.D.s, social workers be M.S.W.s, and that each have several years of past clinical experience. Eight of the thirty-seven clinicians were women. Seven of these were social workers and one a psychologist. All psychiatrists were males. Two were black. Three other blacks (two female and a male) were social workers. No black psychologists participated in the reviews. One psychologist, however, was of Indian origin. All reviewers were judged by screening attorneys to be clear and articulate users of the English language.

*Team Members: How They Become Involved*

Review team members differed in terms of how they initially became involved in the patient review process. Psychiatrists were primarily recruited by Ohio Mental Health officials. Psychologists were split between those contracted by state officials and those approached by colleagues (who had been approached by officials). On the other hand social workers became involved either through their own initiative (that is, reading about the process in the papers and deciding to volunteer) or by the invitation of lawyers for the plaintiffs. Given this differentiation, it is interesting to ask whether the route to involvement was symbolically paired with some notion of stratified professional prestige. Our interviews with the participating professionals indicated that, while other members were unclear about why they were selected, those approached by mental health officials generally attributed their selection to the possession of desirable professional qualities (that is, considerable past experience, laudable credentials, recognition or officership in professional societies). Moreover, several psychiatrists were critical of the role played by patient lawyers in the recruitment process. It was their opinion that recruitment should have been in the sole hands of mental health professionals (like themselves). Inasmuch as the routes to initial involvement varied along disciplinary lines and may also have implied differences in imputed professional prestige, the recruitment process appears to foreshadow the development of important status differentials between team members. This matter and its impact on the review is the subject for a more detailed analysis in process in Chapter 9.

*Professional Orientations of Team Members*

In order to know whether team members had brought a particular clinical or theoretical focus to their diagnostic work, they were asked whether they identified with any particular "school" or professional orientation within their discipline. Half answered that they were eclectic, suggesting that they "use whatever method seems appropriate for an individual patient." Slightly less than a third said that, although they try to fit treatment to individual needs, in figuring out a patient's problems they primarily used somewhat of a psychoanalytic perspective. The remaining clinicians were scattered between perspectives emphasizing the behavioral or learning theory model, insight therapy, or a stress on the role of the self in a psychosocial context. Overall, psychologists and social workers were most diverse in the ascription of self labels, while psychiatrists saw themselves as either eclectic or psychoanalytic.

*Past Experience with "Maximum Security Forensic Patients"*

Approximately two-thirds of the clinicians interviewed believed that they had past experience with the types of patients housed in a setting like Lima State Hospital. Yet, in seeking documentation of the actual nature of their past clinical experiences, it was evident that some team members were much more inclusive than others regarding the notion of past work with similar patients. For instance, some members defined similarity so as to include such diverse groupings as clients of a methodone clinic, the "borderline mentally retarded," or "acute nonhospitalized children." When we recoded answers in terms of actual past experience with forensic patients who were potential candidates for maximum security, the segment of clinicians with actual past experience was reduced to approximately two-fifths. More important, however, were the noticed experiential differences among disciplines. Considerably more psychiatrists (five out of eight) and psychologists (four out of nine) than social workers (two out of twelve) responding to this question were categorized as having had actual past experiences. The importance of this factor awaits our discussion of how members intentionally use such things as displays of past experience in negotiating status and power differentials during actual diagnostic decision-making (Chapter 9).

*Formal Preparation for the Review Process*

The formal preparation of psychiatric team members for the review of Lima State patients was limited to the series of communications (with mental health officials, legal representatives, or colleagues) that prompted their initial involvement, the distribution of copies of the interim court order, and a one-day-long orientation session. During the orientation session, held the day before the review process officially commenced, members were given a simplified guide to the court order and were presented with background information on the hospital, its patients, and their professional mission. The highlight of this orientation session was a discussion of issues involved in the prediction of dangerousness by a panel of "experts," assembled by state mental health officials. Reiterating the wording of the court order this panel suggested that the reviewers' mission was "very clear and easy." The only three questions they had to answer were (1) whether a patient was mentally ill or mentally retarded, (2) whether a patient was an immediate danger to self or others, and (3) whether a patient could be contained in a lesser restrictive environment than Lima State Hospital. According to the expert panel, "All you need to do is say yes or no on each question. It's very simple."

Most team members did not think the issues were as clear as suggested. A flurry of questions were immediately directed to the panel. What about patients categorized as nondangerous because they were on medication? What types of maximum security settings were available outside Lima, and how did these compare with those in Lima? What would happen to and with a patient if a team recommended a release? The panel, however, suggested that the participants were overcomplicating the issues. "Why ask more questions than required?" The psychiatric decision-makers had only to decide on the immediateness of danger. "Now is now," and what happens to a patient in the (nonimmediate) future is beyond the scope of the patient reviewer's mission.

The emphasis on the "immediateness" and "ease" of their predictive task did not satisfy many clinicians. Many, particularly psychiatrists, argued that in order to provide a professional assessment of a patient's likely behavior, they needed to know what circumstances the patient would encounter in the future. Others suggested that they might be legally liable in the future for their "medical" judgments in the present. The court-appointed master of the case attempted to address (or "cool out") these questions by suggesting that members need not worry because most patients will not be released or "put back on the streets," but will simply be transferred to less restrictive, but still supervised, environments. Furthermore, the actual decisions to transfer would be made by the judge, and the role of the teams was only to recommend and advise.

The evaluation task still seemed more complicated to a number of team members. What about "psychological harm"? Shouldn't that be part of the definition of dangerousness? Wasn't "immediateness" a vague concept? How soon was "immediate"? The operational meaning of term after term in the court order began to be challenged. Questions were phrased argumentatively. A kind of tension between the psychiatric and legal perspectives was evident. The categories that members were asked to use were said to be legal terms which constrained the psychiatric practices with which members were professionally most familiar.

After a period of aggressive bantering back and forth, one panel member eventually stated, "Well, of course, we cannot define away your professional judgment." Team members were told that they would have to rely on whatever clinical methods they would ordinarily use and simply see that those were paired with the commitment requirements set by the court. The state of tension was relaxed. Team members asked a few final questions, but without the aggressive posture of those before. Immediately after the discussion, an observer asked the most belligerent of the participants if their questions had been satisfactorily answered. Each explained that up until the panel acknowledged that they still had to rely on their professional judgments they had felt cornered into doing something which seemed unduly constraining. They could answer the legal question, but needed to use their own psychiatric methods. Before the panel's admission of this fact, members had felt that they were being asked to burden themselves with a "legal" methodology for which they were not suited. Once it was perceived that they were given "free reign" to do what they do best, members no longer saw problems with the mission ahead. Most voiced statements of confidence in the upcoming review process.

The tension and tension release described above are indicative of a certain conflict between psychiatric and legal definition of the diagnostic mission. This conflict was also revealed in members' evaluation of the helpfulness of the orientation session and of the court order in preparing for their work. This assessment varied across disciplinary statuses. Most psychiatrists did not find the court order to be of much assistance, and nearly all psychiatrists and psychologists felt that there was little or no benefit to the formal orientation provided them. On the other hand, the majority of social workers found both the order and the orientation helpful. The majority of psychologists also found the order at least somewhat helpful.

These differentiated responses, while interesting, are not entirely unexpected. Research has consistently documented the medical profession's desire to control the processes and consequences of its decision-making. The frequent structural and perceptual designation of psychologists as "forensic experts" may likewise account for their negative evaluation of what they believed to be a nonexpert and disorganized orientation program. The fact that psychologists evaluated the court order more favorably than psychiatrists is perhaps suggestive of psychologists' more formalized approach to diagnostic classification. Unlike psychiatrists, who are taught to rely more heavily on their clinical judgments and past professional experience, psychologists tend to be professionally socialized into the use of more defined or structured approaches to investigating a client's "inner life." In contrast, the more favorable assessments by social workers may reflect their general socialization as structural subordinates (to courts and other formal organizations) and their perceived dependence on other experts (for instructions on what to do and feedback on how they are doing it). Such disciplinary differences will be examined for their impact on the production of particular diagnostic styles and outcomes in the chapters to follow.

## The Lima Patients

In recent years Lima State Hospital has changed its designation as a ''hospital for the criminally insane'' to that of a "forensic psychiatric institution." This change more accurately reflects the plurality of categories constituting its patient population. There were, at the time of the patient reviews, seven general categories of patients at this maximum-security institution. In addition to a small number of "criminally insane," the Lima State population included a large number of penal transfers, persons considered incompetent to stand trial, and psychopathic offenders. Also included in lesser numbers were persons transferred from civil hospitals, those found to be "mentally ill" while on parole, and those committed as "extremely dangerous" by probate courts.

Actually only a small number of its residents are technically classified as the "criminally insane" (not guilty by reason of insanity). Out of 716 resident patients in July of 1974 (two months before the patient reviews), only forty-two were indefinitely committed under Ohio's statute requiring hospitalization following a verdict of not guilty by reason of insanity.[5] On the other hand, the largest groupings of Lima patients were divided between two categories: penal transfers and patients considered incompetent to stand trial. Each category represented about one-third of the hospital population. In July of 1974, Lima State Hospital housed 224 individuals transferred from correctional settings and 214 persons committed for hospitalization until "restored to sufficient reason" so as to be competent to stand trial.[6]

The third-largest category of patients at Lima State Hospital consisted of patients committed under Ohio's version of a sexual psychopath statute. Referred to as Asherman patients (named after the legislator introducing this commitment statute), these persons numbered 148 out of a total of 716 patients in the months immediately prior to the patient reviews. Since Asherman patients are generally believed to represent a special type of patient, most are housed for treatment in a special facility on the grounds of, but not within the main structure of, Lima State Hospital. According to the Asherman statute any offender convicted of specific (primarily sexual) crimes must undergo a psychiatric examination after conviction and before sentencing.[7] If such an examination determines that an individual is mentally ill, mentally retarded, or a psychopathic offender, then the individual may be placed on probation or have a sentence imposed and simultaneously suspended, and thus be committed to a psychiatric facility.

We have previously discussed (in Chapter 2) the unspecific application of terms classifying various mental disorders, particularly the use of the term "psychopathic personality." the vagueness of such terminology has promoted criticism of the Asherman statute. It defines the psychopathic offender as:

Any person who is adjudged to have a psychopathic personality, who exhibits criminal tendencies, and who by reasons thereof is a menace to the public. Psychopathic personality is evidenced by such traits or characteristics inconsistent with the age of such person, as emotional immaturity and instability, impulsive, irresponsive, reckless, and unruly acts expressively self-centered attitude, deficient powers of self-discipline, lack of normal capacity to learn from experience, marked deficiency of normal sense or control.[8]

In addition to the operational vagueness of its definitions, the Asherman statute has also been criticized for being too inclusive and for legislating contradictory philosophies. Besides specifying crimes which mandate a psychiatric examination toward possible commitment, the act provides any trial court with the discretion of referring any defendant convicted of a felony or a misdemeanor, who is thought to be possibly mentally ill, mentally retarded, or psychopathic. The Asherman Act's equivocation between a philosophy of treatment and one of punishment has also been a subject for debate. This equivocation is underlined by a trial court's option to reinstate a patient's original sentence and send him or her to a penal institution at the very point in which it is determined that he or she is recovered or no longer needs the special custody of a state hospital.

The remainder of Lima patients are differentiated among several additional categories. Already mentioned were the indefinitely committed "criminally insane."[9] Also included in the population of Lima patients are persons transferred from civil hospitals on the basis of their alleged dangerousness or disorderly conduct. Although these individuals are not charged with any specific crime, they are housed alongside those under the auspices of various criminal courts. "Thus, for this type of criminally insane patient, there is no criminal conviction (or even complaint), but the label is acquired by transfer to an institution for the criminally insane."[10] A small number of persons found to be mentally ill while on parole or considered dangerous by various local probate courts round out the diverse groupings of patients residing at Lima State Hospital.

*Summary Comments*

In this short chapter we have provided background information on our two main categories of actors: the psychiatrist professionals and the patients they diagnosed. Our intention was to provide the reader with a descriptive sense of actors and their sociolegal status. In the next chapter we shall turn our attention to the actual work of the court-ordered diagnosers and to the manner in which they framed assumptions about their work.

**Notes**

1. "Two Hundred Hear Day-Long Discussion of 'Right to Treatment,' "
*Mental Horizons* (a publication of the Ohio Department of Mental Health and
Mental Retardation) 1, 4 (August): 7.

2. Background data on the legal action and actors behind the court order
were obtained from a series of in-depth interviews with attorneys representing
both the state and the plaintiffs.

3. C. Thomas McCarter, "John Davis' Quest Was for Treatment, But He
Also Fought John Malpass," a paper presented at the Fifth Annual Institute on
Law and Psychiatry, Southern Illinois University, Carbondale, Illinois, Nov. 13,
1974, p. 12.

4. The guidelines were set forth in the interim order: *John Davis et al.*
(plaintiffs) v. *Paul Watkins et al.* (defendants); Order of U.S. District Judge
Nicholas Walinski, No. C. 73-205 in the U.S. District Court for the Northern
District of Ohio Western Division.

5. These figures and others presented hereafter are based upon the Month-
ly Statistical Summary Report, Ohio Department of Mental Health and Mental
Retardation (July 1974), p. 9. This data is summarized in James M. Caulfield,
"Ohio Commitments to the Mentally Ill Offender," *Capital University Law
Review* 4, 1: 1-36.

6. The commitment statutes governing penal transfers and the "incompetent to stand trial" have been the target of criticism by various civil liber-
tarian interests. "Mentally ill" prisoners are administratively transferred from
correctional to mental health institutions. This procedure, without provision
of a separate hearing for the purpose of determining "commitability," is said
to violate a patient's right to due process. This situation is made more problematic by the fact that many patient/inmates remain indefinitely committed
at Lima State Hospital in considerable excess of the time of their maximum
penal sentence. Patients ruled incompetent to stand trial have experienced
much the same difficulty. Technically never convicted of a crime, such patients
have often been involuntarily confined for periods equal to and in excess of
what would potentially have been the maximum sentence potentially imposed
if convicted. Although many jurisdictions have recently followed the Supreme
Court decision in *Jackson* v. *Indiana* by statutorily limiting commitment for
incompetency to a maximum of 180 days, Ohio's response has relied instead
on an executive order of a former director of its Department of Mental Health
and Mental Retardation. The uncodified nature of this response has been questioned on the grounds that it provides no statutory safeguard protecting a
patient's rights. Despite such criticism, however, "incompetency" and "penal
transfers" were the two major categories by which patients were classified at
the time of the Lima patient reviews.

For an extended discussion of these matters, see James M. Caulfield, "Ohio Commitments."

7. The so-called Asherman Statute is contained under the Ohio Revised Code 2945.25.

8. Ohio Revised Code 2947.24(B) (Page Supp. 1972). Also excerpted in Caulfield, p. 28.

9. The failure to distinguish between insanity at the time of a crime and the posttrial continuance of presumed insanity has brought about considerable criticism of this particular pathway to commitment.

10. Henry Steadman and Joseph Cocozza, *Careers of the Criminally Insane: Excessive Social Control of Deviance* (Lexington, Mass.: Lexington Books, 1974).

# 6

## Framing the Psychiatric Mission: Clinicians' Purposes-at-Hand and Assumptions About Diagnostic Categories

*Is the patient well enough to leave the hospital? [T]he knowledge necessary to answer this question is not readily available for us in a highly rational, calculable, and predictable manner. How, then, do staff . . . govern their own decisions? Obviously, they must operate within some framework of standards which provides* structure *for the decision-making process. It is this structure that provides legitimacy to the staff decisions. Again, staff decisions cannot be made without standards or criteria, nor can the standards be "pulled out of a hat." . . . The standards must have some credibility, be it relevant knowledge or "masking" beliefs.*

> Robert Perrucci, *Circle of Madness* (Englewood Cliffs, N.J.: 1974), pp. 149-150)

The manner in which people frame definitions of what it is that they are doing, and how it is that that which is being done should be done, is of great importance in shaping the end-product of social interaction. In this chapter we shall consider the way that psychiatric review team members frame the purposes of their mission—their purposes-at-hand. We shall also consider the manner in which they frame assumptions about the definitions of various legal questions and clinical categories. The manner in which members interactionally approach each other, patients, and the legal actors to which they report is directly influenced by the ways that these framings are accomplished. As such, this chapter may be read as a prelude to our analysis of the diagnosis-producing interactions discussed in the chapters to follow.

### Members' Purposes-at-Hand

Whether one is attending a dull classroom lecture, robbing a bank, or caressing the face of a sweetheart, one's purpose-at-hand, the intentional direction of consciousness, is often multi-focused.[1] Although actors may single out a particular goal as the avowed objective of social interaction, several ends may be realized in one sequence of human behavior. The fact that these ends may be, at one time, anticipated or unanticipated, compatible or incompatible, should not concern us at this point. Clearly, a simultaneity of lived projects, a multiplicity of purpose-at-hand, is a fact of everyday human experience. The anxious student, the psychoanalyzed bank robber, or the self-gratified lover provide evidence of this experience. The student may sit out the boring lecture both for the purposes of salvaging a bit of knowledge and fulfilling the attendance requirements of the professor. Both purposes, not one alone, may be said to guide social interaction in this instance. So may the robber empty the bank vault both for money and as a "manly" display of aggression. Likewise, the lover may gently touch the loved one, realizing at one and the same time the act of loving and the engenderment of being loved.

As with the actors being described above, the actions of patient review team members appeared to be guided by more than one purpose-at-hand. Two general purposes are of particular relevance to the present analysis. The first was simply to accomplish the diagnostic mission set forth by the court. Team members acted in order to "make sense" out of a patient, his or her record, talk, and behavior. This "sense-making" was accompanied by a second purpose. Team members also worked to accomplish a situated identity as professionals. Not only did members work to obtain personal knowledge about the status of a patient; they also endeavored to display publicly that knowledge in such a way that it would be recognized as valid, objective, and expert by others. Their purposes-at-hand, in other words, included both "making sense" and "appearing expertly sensible."

"Making sense" out of a patient involved a variety of interactional strategies which are described in the following three chapters. The purpose of these was to establish (that is, construct, stabilize, and defend) identitites for patients as types of persons. "Appearing expertly sensible" also involved a variety of interactional strategies. The purpose of these was to establish identities for team members as types of persons with access to privileged knowledge. It involves the selective presentation of themselves as experts. The audience for this presentation included other team members and the administrative-legal community which commissioned their work.

Many of the "appearing expert" strategies were nonverbal. They included the preoccupied pondering or rapid note construction of team members unsure of their impressions concerning a patient, but unwilling to have other members "see" their unsuredness. They included the demonstrative gestures of a psychiatrist flicking a match before a patient's eyes in order to display for others his insight into the nature of a patient's perceptual alertness. They included the "reflective stroking" of a beard by one clinician and the "summary winking" of another (indicative that a diagnostic decision had been reached.) They included the sensitive but firm ushering in of an elderly and disoriented patient. All of these gestures spoke a message of professionality. All were indicative that members were conducting interaction in an expert manner.

Even more important were the written-language strategies. These were of particular relevance to the legal audience which would typically have access to only what members had written about patients. In appearing expert, members did not make general observations about the human behavior they observed. They "discovered" syndromes and symptoms of clinical significance that the nonexpert would simply bypass. The mutual display of such specialized language is presented in the following excerpted exchange between a psychiatrist and a psychologist.

Excerpt 6-1. From Patient Review 442, Team D

(410)  *Psychiatrist*:  He showed good control. He'd get his affect up and then he'd get it throttled down again. And he was irritated by some of the things on the unit. And he certainly seemed, you know, he didn't go completely out of control. He didn't disintegrate or disorganize when he did this sort of thing.

(411)  *Psychologist*:  I got the feeling there was some paranoid anger coming out towards the end, when he was talking about his treatment.

(412)  *Psychiatrist*:  Well, it's unclear that . . . .

(413)  *Psychologist*:  I don't mean to insist he's delusional.

(414)  *Psychiatrist*:  Yeah, right.

(415)  *Psychologist*:  I was just saying he has, I think, paranoid and schizoid features to his personality.

Note the technical or even mechanistic language employed by the psychiatrist in line 410. "He'd get his affect up." "He didn't disintegrate or disorganize." Such language categorizes the patient. It also facilitates the presentation of an expert identity for the physician. In this regard, the quick diagnostic realignment by the psychologist in line 413 is of particular interest. The psychologist appears desirous of complimenting rather than challenging the professional posture of the psychiatrist. Line 412, however, appears to be heard as a line of possible contradiction to the presentation of an "expert" identity through language use. This contradiction is interactionally warded off in the subsequent exchanges.

The importance of appearing expertly professional is documented in numerous other observations. A useful mechanism for one member to gain a negotiating advantage over another is to call into question the other's professional displays. In one decision-making sequence a psychiatrist and psychologist, who disagreed with the diagnosis of a particular social worker, asked this dissident member to evaluate her own emotional involvement in the case. The message was clear. What team members were bargaining with was the situated professional identities of each other. In another instance. a psychiatrist disagreeing with the judgments of his fellow team members reminded them not to confuse documented fact with speculative theory. A psychologist haggling over a diagnosis with a social worker was quick to point out that concern with the question of dangerousness was an inappropriate framework for considering psychopathic offenders. In each case, the invocation of a "professional rule" or "expert norm" was contextually deployed so as to block a member's situated attainment of "expert identity." Such identity is, after all, dependent on the recognition and response of others. Observations of its ongoing establishment and defense lead to the inference that this was a major purpose-at-hand for team members acting together.

The use of specialized language is an important vehicle for establishing an expert identity. In the following excerpt, a psychiatrist has become bothered by minor terminological challenges of the team's social worker. By employing and explaining language "beyond" the domain of the social worker's knowledge, the psychiatrist is able to establish his preeminently expert identity and challenge the expertness of his diagnostic competitor. This use of "expert-appearing" language facilitates a supportive coalition between the psychiatrist and psychologist. The social worker must either come back into line or have his professional status implicitly discredited.

Excerpt 6-2. From Patient Review 363, Team L

(113)  *Psychiatrist*: Charges—"incest." One to ten. Diagnosis—sexual deviation? Now, I don't argue with that. For gosh sakes! Wait while I make a notation on that.

(114)  *Psychologist*: I don't either.

(115)  *Social Worker*: What was that?

(116)  *Psychiatrist*: Pedophilia—meaning he goes after children. From pediatrics. I wouldn't go for that.

(117)  *Psychologist*: What would you say? Inadequate personality?

(118)  *Psychiatrist*: Why, certainly I would; that adult stress reaction, and I would say inept personality, and then the sexual deviation is explaining the act he committed by not the reason.

(119)  *Psychologist*: No.

(120)  *Social Worker*: But he did it only with his daughter.

(121)  *Psychiatrist*: Well, that's right. Special readjustment to stress and it wouldn't have mattered if he was fifteen or thirteen or fourteen or any other age.

(122)  *Psychologist*: Right.

As important as it was to appear professional before each other, it was equally important for members to establish the appearance of expertise before the legal audience to which they reported. Interactional work was performed to transform feelings into findings and perceive states of affairs into expert opinions. A show of general uncertainty or confusion was frequently blocked.

This insulation of "what goes on," in favor of what members wanted outside audiences to see, is illustrated in the following excerpt. Note the situated evocation of a "don't publicly express confusion rule." In this instance it was situationally evoked by one member when another member, perplexed by the complexity of a case, was perceived as endangering the team's purpose of "appearing expertly sensible."

Excerpt 6-3. From Patient Review 113, Team A

(The team is making its final recommendations. It has spent considerable time trying to make sense out of a patient's jumbled legal record. The excerpt begins with the comments of one of this team's two psychologists. It is the social worker who is dictating the final report into a tape recorder.)

(801)    *Psychologist A*:  We need to recommend that someone review the legal confusion.

(802)    *Psychologist B*:  Yeah, and the confusion of the hospital.

(803)    *Social Worker* (dictating):  This team is confused and unable to determine the present legal status of . . . .

(804)    *Psychologist B*:  No. Don't say we're confused, even if we are.

(805)    *Social Worker*:  Oh, OK. What if I say we were unable from the record to determine the basis . . . .

(806)    *Psychologist A*:  Right. It's the legal record that's the problem.

(807)    *Psychiatrist*:  And we could say that there's unclarity also in the hospital record.

(808)    *Social Worker* (dictating again):  This team was unable from the legal record to determine the basis for the patient's continued commitment at Lima State Hospital. It should be noted that there was considerable unclarity in this record and in the hospital record as well.

In the preceding excerpt, the team negotiates the wording of a report so that it is clear that it is the record and not their expertness which is challengeable. The following comments by a participating psychiatrist reveal a similar strategy. The "unrealistic" legal demands of the court are believed to jeopardize the expertise of the patient reviewers. If final decisions are worded in the "clear-cut" language, psychiatric professionals may too readily be proved wrong. Their expertness would be potentially discreditable. The preservation of expert identity requires more discretionary vagueness. The introduction of this vagueness through a highly specialized vocabulary is explained in the following statement.

Excerpt 6-4. From Psychiatrist Interview

Our concern was that it was a responsibility to say—as I saw this individual today he was perfectly fine and we saw no signs of potential danger. But they were asking us clear-cut. And when we asked what about if they act out tomorrow they said, "We're not interested in tomorrows. We're interested in today." Well, that's narrowing down. Which is, you know, not really what we do in practice. If a patient is in the hospital, he is medicated. He's improved and so on. Fine. He might act out two or three days later again. But today if you interview and find no [signs], I'm not saying this individual is not dangerous. I never do this. We say he is potentially dangerous, although controlled at this time. You know, you never leave the door that wide open. Not with these cases.

But we were asked to do that. And we were concerned and we asked the question—what responsibility do we have when we find them totally fine and then ten days from now he acts out? And especially the individual on medication. . . . This is why we always, in our recommendation, put down "we feel at this time he's in remission, well controlled, but should remain on medication because . . . they are psychotic patients."

The concern with one's situated expert identity is a "purpose-at-hand" which temporally coexists with team members' efforts to make sense out of and diagnose patients. Members appear sensitive to the consequences of their "sense-making" as it impacts upon their appearances as expertly sensible professionals. This sensitivity manifests itself in various nonverbal and verbal displays, particularly in the formulation and articulation of a specialized professional vocabulary. The interactional strategies accompanying this second "purpose-at-hand" should be kept in mind in subsequently considering the various practices that members used to cognitively and publicly categorize patients.

### Members' Assumptions about Review Categories

Judgments about patients were significantly influenced by the manner in which psychiatric professionals framed assumptions about the meaning of this or that clinical category. These assumptions functioned as the definitional parameters or operating definitions within which teams negotiated decisions about mental illness or retardation, dangerousness, the need for maximum security, incompetence to stand trial, and continued placement within a treatment unit for "psychopathic offenders." Before fully appreciating the role of these definitional assumptions, one must understand the nature of the diagnostic judgments mandated by the court.

The federal court directed the Lima patient review teams to make several types of clinical judgments. Technically the nature of these judgments was to vary with the legal status of each patient.[2] In practice the judgmental activity fell into three categories. The first included judgments about the mental illness or retardation, dangerousness, and need for maximum security for those transferred from either penal or civil institutions, for those committed directly from parole, probation, or probate court settings, for those found not guilty by reason of insanity, and for those who remain hospitalized after the expiration of their maximum criminal sentences. The second centered on judgments about a patient's appreciation of his or her criminal charges and whether or not he or she could assist an attorney in preparing a legal defense. This category was applicable only for those patients previously found incompetent to stand trial. The third and final category paired judgments about mental illness or retardation with those concerning whether an individual was a psychopathic offender and could benefit by further treatment in a special unit for patients committed under Ohio's Ascherman (or sexual psychopath) Act.

While decisions about a particular clinical label varied with the legal category of a given patient, in general, team members had to decide upon the applicability of six distinct diagnostic categories. The assumptions which informed the use of these categories are discussed in the following pages.

### Assumptions about Mental Illness

Patient review teams assumed that the term mental illness was the functional equivalent of psychosis. The presence of mental illness appeared dependent on the recognition of one of three psychotic symptoms. These included the inability to coherently order one's conversation, the manifestation of delusional thinking, or the manifestation of hallucinations. In the absence of these symptoms, members assumed that a patient was not behaving as a mentally ill person at the present time.

All but a few patients reviewed for mental illness were found to be either still mentally ill or mentally ill but in a state of remission. The fact that patients were not believed to be behaving as mentally ill persons was not a sufficient reason for team members to state officially that they were not mentally ill. A clear-cut statement as to the absence of mental illness emerged under all but three limited conditions. Patients were so categorized only if: (1) their past record had no allegation of past psychosis; (2) they were so old that future aberrations in behavior could be attributed to "incursions of senescence"; or (3) the decisions mandated by the court (that is, a judgment as to competency to stand trial) could be made without any reference to mental illness.

If none of the preceding conditions was present and patients were still perceived to have not behaved as mentally ill persons, teams appeared to operate on the assumption that they could not (or should not) be clear-cut in noting the absence of illness. Although a patient acted appropriately and conversed competently, it was generally stated that he or she was still mentally ill but "in remission" or "in good control" at the present time. In a few cases a statement that a patient was not mentally ill was immediately followed by a seemingly contradictory statement suggesting that the person was actually ill, but in remission.

The cautious use of "remission" terminology could possibly be explained by team members' theoretical assumptions about the continuity of mental illness. If a patient's past record suggested previous episodes of psychosis, the best that team members would say was that he or she was in remission or good control in the present. Implied was the notion that the illness might reemerge in the future. This operative assumption about the use of the "remission" label is compatible with that body of psychiatric literature which suggests that a serious mental disease (for example, schizophrenia) never entirely disappears. The disease is said to be only more or less controlled at the present time.

While the theoretical assumption about the continuity of illness may have guided some members' judgmental practices, it is also likely that a practical assumption about the consequences of their decisions was operative as well. This observation is compatible with our previous discussion regarding members' concern with the way others assessed their appearance as experts. The true test of their expertness would come in time. Teams interviewed patients at but one interval in history. If a patient was assessed as not mentally ill in the present but manifested a psychotic break at some point in the future, a team's judgments would certainly be open to question. Of course, it could always be reasoned that the illness had not emerged or had not been induced at the time of a team's assessment of the patient. This line of defense, however, is less tenable if others, in previous times, had noted the presence of illness. Why had other professionals, but not the review teams, seen the signs of a patient's mental disease? Under this condition, the substance of a diagnostic judgment has a direct bearing on members' accomplishment of expert identities. As such, teams' decisions are carefully worded. If the past record indicated the presence of previous psychotic episodes, members were careful to include remission terminology in describing patients who were not behaving as mentally ill persons in the present.

The exceptions to the use of guarded remission terminology occurred in situations where the consequences of making clear-cut statements about the absence of illness were less problematic. Some patients were so old that future bizarre behaviors could be interpreted as "incursions of senescence" rather than as mental illness. Such an interpretation would defend a team's expert judgment about the lack of illness. As such, it is interesting to note that several of the small number of cases in which teams appeared to make clear-cut judgments about the absence of mental illness occurred with very elderly and often physically deteriorating patients. Yet, despite supposed clear-cutness, these judgments were not accompanied by suggestions that patients be released outright. Statements were rendered somewhat less "clear-cut" by additional recommendations for continued care "in less confined" situations.

A second condition which lessened the problematic consequences of stating that a person was not mentally ill involved cases in which the review teams were not asked to make judgments about mental illness per se. The major example, of course, concerned cases in which members were to decide competency to stand trial. Teams could make cursory judgments about mental illness which had little consequence for the maintenance of their identities as experts. Their responsibility was formally limited to the questions they were asked to answer. Statements about mental illness were made only to the degree that they would impact on the ability to appreciate criminal charges or assist in one's defense. Hence, teams occasionally volunteered statements about the absence of mental illness in situations where it mattered little or had little consequence. In situations where the consequences mattered, where teams' expert judgments were on the line, teams were much more cautious. They couched their diagnostic statements in language like that presented below.

Excerpt 6-5. From Final Report of Team L

As the patient was interviewed, he appeared to be in good contact with reality. Although somewhat constricted in affect, he did answer questions appropriately. He is obviously psychotic, but in good control at this time.

Excerpt 6-6. From Final Report of Team B

He is oriented for time, place, and person and shows no evidence of memory impairment for either recent or remote past. There is no disturbance of thought content either in the form of delusional ideation or hallucinations manifest at this time. His judgment, reality testing, insight appear to be fairly well intact. . . . Patient is not considered to be mentally ill at this time. His psychosis seems to be in remission.

Assumptions about coherent conversation, and the manifestations of either delusions or hallucinations, operated as guides in the recognition of present mental illness. Assumptions about the continuity of mental illness and the consequences of particular diagnostic wordings operated as guides for the formulation of statements about the absence or remission of mental illness when these psychotic symptoms were believed not to be present. One additional set of assumptions further guided teams in formulating statements about the presence of mental illness. These were assumptions about the meaning of a patient's medication.

Since most patients were divided between being categorized as either presently mentally ill or as in remission from mental illness, it would seem that the latter grouping represented a body of persons who were perceived as better off. This distinction is true for most patients but not for all patients. Because of certain assumptions that several teams made about the use of psychotropic medication, some patients, who manifested none of the assumed characteristics of mental illness, were classified as being mentally ill simply because they were on medication. Their behaviors were essentially no different from those which would lead other teams to classify patients as being in remission (or in the three limited conditions as being "not mentally ill"). What was different were certain teams' assumptions about the relationship between being mentally ill and being on medication.

Many teams appeared to treat the use of medication as a variable that existed somewhat independently of a person's mental illness. Teams often stated that a patient was in "satisfactory remission" and could be transferred to a less restrictive environment, without ever mentioning the fact that the patient was on medication. Other teams would state that the patient was in remission while on medication. In both instances the "positive" fact of remission would be entered into the patient's permanent record. This fact would inform future reviewers and agents of social control of a patient's progress toward normality. A few teams, however, upon noting the use of medication, felt obliged to render a formal diagnosis that the patient was still mentally ill. Although it was believed that the patient did not act mentally ill, it was reasoned that since he or she was on psychotropic medication, he or she must be mentally ill. Why else would one be on medication? On this assumption the "negative" fact of continued mental illness would be entered into the patient's permanent record.

The inference of continued mental illness from continued medication represents a particular problem for patients with hopes of freeing themselves from what Perrucci has called the institutionalized "circle of madness." This circularity was actually described by one team as a kind of "Catch-22" situation in which the patient's good behavior (on medication) was taken as evidence of the patient's real illness (and hence, need for further medication).

Excerpt 6-7. From Patient Review 71, Team J

(The team has already formulated a version of its final decision in which they stated that the patient "is not overtly mentally ill at this time," while noting that "there's a strong suggestion that he has been in the past." In reviewing this decision, the issue of medication arises. Notice how the team arrives at an operating definition about this matter which changes its original decision.)

(671)  *Psychologist*:  OK, is he mentally ill?

(672)  *Psychiatrist*:  No.

(673)  *Psychologist*:  Yes, but he's —

(674)  *Psychiatrist*:  It's tough.

(675)  *Psychologist*:  Oh, yes.

(676)  *Social Worker*:  OK, now you've forced me back into the testing situation again, which I thought was resolved. Uh, OK, well then, but you're talking in terms of continuing medication, and continued treatment, right?

(677)  *Psychiatrist*:  Yeah.

(678)  *Social Worker*:  But you're saying he's not mentally ill?

(679)  *Psychiatrist*:  As long as he continues his medication.

(680) *Social Worker*: But if he's not mentally ill he doesn't, you know, Why, why does he need this?

(681) *Psychiatrist*: That's the Catch-22. . . .

(682) *Social Worker*: Yeah. Now is it? Yes. He's mentally ill, uh. . . .

(683) *Psychologist*: [The social worker] is suggesting the model that if a person needs treatment, then he must be mentally ill.

(684) *Social Worker*: Yeah, but yeah, which is more in terms of a legal model rather than, you know, uh, uh, a mental health model, but it's the, you know, it is the board that sent us in here, and they don't, and, you know, I'm saying from the legal mind, you know, it leaves them to think, you know, you're going to treat this man, but he's not sick, uh, you know, it sounds. . . .

(685) *Psychiatrist*: Well, let's say that he is. . . .

(686) *Social Worker*: And that he's not psychotic but that he's mentally ill.

(687) *Psychiatrist*: . . . He's not psychotic. His mental illness is in a state of resolution. He's on medication. He no longer needs a maximum-security institution. He could be managed by another program in the community.

(688) *Psychologist*: But if you say his mental illness is in a state of resolution, that might be confusing to them.

(689) *Psychiatrist*: It isn't to me, it may be to them.

(690) *Psychologist*: I know, but, uh, I think they want a fairly clear-cut answer . . . (unclear).

(691) *Social Worker*: Well, I kind of buy that; OK, maybe is this what we're saying? That he is not mentally ill because he's on the medication and, you know, so forth. I . . . I . . . to me that makes sense. Yeah, uh, that's why I agreed a while ago, I guess. That makes sense.

(692) *Psychiatrist*: This is an enigma that's plagued everybody for years, because there's a guy that I testified on three times, that's committed two murders, and he gets in, he takes medication, he's perfectly well, as long as he maintains his medication he's fine, but then he gets thrown out of the cell and becomes dangerous.

(693) *Social Worker*: Yeah, under the medication I guess theoretically he is. . . .

(694) *Psychologist*: You know when he throws up when he doesn't get medication it says he has to be on it. There's some suggestion that he wants to be identified as a patient, but you know, there's something wrong. . . .

(695) *Psychologist*: How much. . .?

(696) *Psychiatrist*: Thirty-eight mgs per day.

(697) *Psychologist*: That's another interpretation of his throwing up. It's that he wants treatment, he wants to be identified as having something wrong with him, and, uh . . . maybe that makes him hard to live with too, and . . . by himself (unclear). But he didn't want to in here.

(698)  *Psychiatrist*: What's the date of, oh, you've got the dates of the murder of his mother and everything, so we can dictate back. OK, I'll bring together that he's mentally ill, but he's in a state of remission with the medication, I can put that in a quote, or can I?

(699)  *Psychologist*: Yeah. Sure.

The psychiatrist in the excerpt above states that he'll "bring together that he's mentally ill, but in a state of remission with the medication." This conclusion, prompted by a particular assumption about medication use, is considerably different from the conclusion that "he is not overtly mentally ill" with which the team began its discussion. The summary paragraph of the team's final report (brought together by the psychiatrist) states simply that "[the patient] is mentally ill." It is this fact, not the negotiated transcripted reasoning in excerpt 6-7, which will be passed on in the patient record. Hence, by virtue of a varying assumption about medication, patients with similar behavioral displays were provided with different diagnostic conclusions.

### Assumptions about Mental Retardation

Teams appeared to assume that two steps were necessary in order for an individual to be classified as mentally retarded. The first was that the patient's record state that he or she was retarded, had a low IQ, or manifested other signs of impaired intelligence. The second was that the patient demonstrate inadequate intellectual functioning in the interview setting.

If a record suggested retardation and team members "recognized" inadequate intellectual functioning it was assumed that the patient was, in fact, retarded. Other than asking a patient to perform a few basic arithmetic calculations and perhaps name a few presidents and state capitals, team members did not ordinarily conduct independent tests for retardation or developmental disabilities.

Excerpt 6-8. From Psychiatrist Interview

There were guys that had no insights into their behavior. They were pretty stereotyped. They just kept saying the same thing over and over and over again. These were also the people who are retarded.

Through interviewing, members either confirmed or modified a previous diagnosis of mental retardation. They did not totally reject such previous assessments. Occasionally a record indicated that a patient was retarded and yet the person responded adequately to questions, showed some insights, demonstrated a minimal use of mathematics, and revealed no loss of memory. In such instances members appeared to doubt the classification of the individual as retarded.

They suggested, instead, that he or she showed signs of being in the general "range of mental retardation" or being "borderline mentally retarded." The use of this modified terminology disqualified retardation as being related to a patient's particular social or legal problems. It did not, however, place teams in the situation of totally rejecting or contradicting a previous professional opinion. In effect, teams were declaring mental retardation to be an irrelevant issue for certain patients, without having to present any specialized evidence for this assertion. The potential consequences of a past diagnosis (that is, a possible emphasis on the problematic nature of retardation) were erased. On the other hand, the general direction of a past diagnosis (possibly based on more specific testing than that performed by review teams) was preserved.

## Assumptions about Incompetence to Stand Trial

Members' assumptions about the meaning of this category were generally very close to those mandated by the legal statutes. The exception to this involved one team which consistently skirted questions concerning the appreciation of charges and ability to assist one's attorney. This team focused instead on questions of mental illness, dangerousness, and need for maximum security. Most teams, however, assumed that their task, for patients in this category, was more limited than for patients in other categories. Operating definitions of competency appeared to focus on two things. The first was whether a patient could verbally tell the story of his or her "allegedly criminal event" in such a manner that team members heard it as coherent and reality oriented. The second concerned whether a patient seemed to understand where he or she presently stood in the criminal justice process and whether the individual had a realistic sense of what a trial might involve.

In considering competency members did not assume that signs of mental illness necessarily precluded an individual from going to trial. Only aspects of mental illness which prohibited a patient from appreciating the situation and seriousness of an alleged crime or blocked participation in his or her defense were viewed as relevant to mandated psychiatric decisions in this area. Other aspects of mental illness were inquired into and often included as additional items on a team's final report. As typified in the following excerpt, however, other aspects of mental illness were not believed to affect a specific decision about competency.

Excerpt 6-9. From Final Report of Team J, case 331

There is a strong paranoid component. He feels he has been misused. However, his reality-testing appears to be relatively intact. His thought processes are logical, coherent, and clear. For purposes of this examination, the examiners do feel that he is competent to stand trial: that he can assist his attorney meaningfully in his defense and that he is able to understand the nature and consequences of his act.

The examiners recognize the potential problems because he is still paranoid toward the remaining lawyer in his case. While aware of this, they think it is beyond the scope of this particular examination to consider that issue.

## Assumptions about Dangerousness

In considering dangerousness, review teams were instructed to determine whether there was an extreme likelihood that a patient will do immediate harm to self or others. Several assumptions operated to make this working definition more specific. The first of these assumptions narrowed the notion of harm. Only those behaviors which were considered as "harmful to life" were assumed to be dangerous.

Excerpt 6-10. From Psychologist Interview

Dangerousness is danger to life. . . . My personal definition of snatching a purse or you know, maybe minor physical hurt—I would not consider that real dangerousness. That could happen if a person loses his temper. But when the life is threatened or a very serious physical injury, I would consider that dangerous. Even, I think, in my definition, probably raping I would not consider that very dangerous. Its bad, but I don't consider this dangerous to life.

The restriction of dangerousness to life-threatening behaviors was typical of the definition of nearly all team members. Several mentioned forcible rape, along with murder, as examples of dangerous behaviors. Most commonly, however, it was believed that sexual assaults that were not accompanied by serious personal physical injury were not to be categorized as dangerous. This assumption is revealed in the following final evaluation statements. In noting this definitional restriction, it should be remembered that most "sex offenders" were hospitalized as "sexual psychopaths" and (when believed dangerous) could be retained in a maximum-security setting by criteria other than a statement about the immediacy of their harm to others.[3]

Excerpt 6-11. From Final Evaluation Report of Team B

He is considered to have the capability for repeating, almost immediately, the sexual offenses for which he was charged [sexual molestation of young girls]. But he is not considered to be dangerously assaultive, in that it is not felt that he would be likely to kill. It is, therefore, the opinion of this examining team that this patient is not in need of continued hospitalization in a maximum-security facility.

A second assumption regarding dangerousness was that it was the most difficult of the predictive tasks mandated for the review teams. The following comments are typical of members' beliefs about this issue.

Excerpt 6-12. Excerpt from Psychiatrist Interview

I don't think we're able to spell out what they mean by dangerousness. I think that so difficult. I found it difficult to predict if someone was going to be dangerous, especially when a person had only committed one crime, never had a history of violent behavior, and was behaving well in the hospital.

Although the task was generally viewed as difficult, members expressed guarded confidence that their predictions were reasonably accurate and that they had generally employed the best criteria available. Members often expressed a particular confidence that they were at least able to predict those who would not be dangerous. As stated by one psychiatrist:[4]

Excerpt 6-13. From Psychiatrist Interview

The APA's task force on predicting dangerousness came to the conclusion that you can be just about effective by flipping a coin. . . . We're being asked to do the impossible. . . . I don't think that it's so impossible. It may be impossible in one direction more than in another. It may be impossible to predict accurately everybody who's going to be violent, but I think that you can have some degree of predictability about people who you feel are relatively safe to turn loose. So, for example, I think we were able to come upon many people [for whom] we had the feeling this guy doesn't have to be locked up.

A third assumption about dangerousness involved the criteria teams used to recognize the likelihood for inflicting immediate harm. In nearly all cases, a past history of violence was an assumed prerequisite for viewing a patient as dangerous.

Excerpt 6-14. From Social Worker Interview

In terms of what occurred between [sic] the three of us, I think it's accurate to say that a person would have had to act in a violent fashion, where he would have had to physically harm someone for us to think of him in terms of being dangerous. If that hadn't happened in the past, we didn't blame him as such.

A past history of violence was generally constructed through a survey of a patient's record. Team members cited a number of things within that record which were routinely examined for signs of dangerousness. These included the description of criminal offenses, the record of a fighting or an assaultive incident within the hospital, and the record of times that a patient was placed in seclusion or in restraints. Also considered was a noted shift in a patient's behavior in relation to shifts in medication.

The assumed necessity of a history of violent behavior was modified by two qualifiers. First, most teams weighed recent violence more significantly than that in the distant past. Just how distant the past had to be before a violent act was seen as irrelevant to a present prediction was, however, a judgment which varied across teams and between patients. One team mentioned that a previous man-slaughter incident was unimportant because for the last twenty years the patient had manifested no violence. Another used a ten-year period as a similar yard-stick. Still another stated that the history of a patient's ward behavior for the previous two years was the best indicator of potential dangerousness.

A second qualifier to the assumed necessity of past violence occurs in cases where teams noted the presence of "dangerous delusions." Such delusions were most frequently said to represent paranoid constructions in which patients had much self-investment. It was believed that patients who manifested such psychotic symptoms were likely to act out violently in order to defend their rigid worlds of "unreality." Such delusions were often assumed to be predictive of dangerousness independent of previous behavioral histories.

Excerpt 6-15. From Final Evaluation Report, Team C

She believes that the Mafia, as well as her mother, brother, and sister-in-law are out to kill her by the use of odorless and tasteless poison. Indeed, she states that these people have gotten to the attendants, who then tried to kill her by overdosing her on medicine . . . .

In summary, [the patient] is actively delusional at this time, and the previous diagnosis of schizophrenia, paranoid type, still holds . . . . In reference to the question of dangerousness to others, [the patient] has never been assaultive to anyone although she is often argumentative . . . . However, the investment of her delusional system is seen as so great that she might strike out at anybody who tries to disrupt it . . . . This is a mentally ill woman [paranoid schizophrenia] who has the potential of being dangerous to others. It is suggested that she be retained in Lima.

Qualifiers related to "recency" and "dangerous delusions" modify the use of past violence as a criterion for predicting dangerousness. Past violence was treated as a necessary, but not sufficient, condition in the determination of dangerousness. Teams also made a fourth assumption. It was assumed that the truly dangerous individual would reveal his or her "lack of control" or "lack of ego strength" in the course of an interview. Of course, "uncontrolled impulsivity" could be inferred from a record of repeated violent offenses. In fact, one team relied almost exclusively on the past record, even in cases where patients appeared to be presently cooperative, intact, and had not evidenced violent or disruptive behaviors for an extended period of time.[5] Most teams, however, recognized that records were occasionally incomplete or inaccurate[6] and that they told but an abstract account of incidents that were sometimes situationally based or engendered.[7] Teams thus relied on patients' own accountings of their violence as key elements in assessing the likelihood of immediate dangerousness.

Excerpt 6-16. From Psychiatrist Interview

By looking at the history we could see the repetitiveness, the pattern that was established. And what came through in our own assessment of him in direct interviewing was how he operated, how he exhibited. How he came across. Did we get the feeling that this man was about to blow up or did we feel he had some controls?"

Excerpt 6-17. From Social Worker Interview

We looked at past behaviors. We looked at what it was he did that was called dangerous. . . . Then [in interview] we asked the patient direct questions about possible harm he's done to himself or others, and if he ever thought about anything like this. . . . How does the person handle it when he gets angry; what does he do; what thoughts and fantasies does he have; what were the circumstances if he did strike out at someone? We always got the patient's point of view on the past behavior.

The assessment of a patient's self-control was clearly assumed to be the central element in an interview to determine dangerousness. In the stress of rapid questioning about past and future violence it was believed that patients would reveal the degree to which they were in control of any aggressive impulses. Often, teams applied deliberate pressure and provocation through an aggressive interview technique referred to as "stressing." As one psychiatrist indicated, this technique is believed to uncover whether "the individual is so mentally affected that he cannot use restraints."

Excerpt 6-18. From Psychiatrist Interview

. . . The thing is . . . the amount of control they have in the interview . . . . We did stress them. We thought that was definitely necessary. We guys would shoot questions from the side and occasionally some buts, you know, a few of the fellows would jump up and, you know, some of the crazier ones would go: "I know karate, and you better watch it. I can kill."

Excerpt 6-19. From Psychiatrist Interview

[In the stressed interview] we looked at what was the capacity of the patient to commit an act of violence . . . . We tried to see how imminent or what kind of provocation would trigger this kind of behavior; and how loose his control was; and how remote the situation was; and how much maturation had taken place since the last act of violence.

The four assumptions discussed so far (that dangerousness meant life-threatening, that dangerousness implied a most difficult decision, that dangerousness required a past history of violence, that dangerousness is revealed in the stress of interviewing) were manifested by each of the review teams. Teams also varied in making more specialized or idiosyncratic assumptions. It was already mentioned that one team appeared to place a greater emphasis on the past record. Another team focused more on a patient's ability to express insight into past deeds of violence. Another paid more attention to a patient's verbalization of his or her dreams and fantasies. Another believed the results of psychological testing were very helpful and complained that these were not uniformly available for all patients. Still, another team paid considerable attention to signs of dangerousness that it believed to be present in a patient's "repressed anger." According to that team's psychologist, a patient who "could not express anger" was assumed to be potentially dangerous and explosive." This member cited a case in which the team asked a patient what it felt like to be a bastard. The patient's passive, nonemotive response ("I don't like it") was assumed to be a cue that anger and potential violence were simmering within. This assumption was also expressed by another member of the same review team, who stated that "I have a feeling if people, if they lash out with very, very little provocation, that there must be so much anger that they are likely to murder somebody or kill somebody, or do very real harm."

Another team's idiosyncratic assumption is expressed in the following excerpt. While this assumption cannot be generalized to all teams, it provides additional evidence of the significance of members' operating definitions about particular diagnostic categories.

Excerpt 6-20. From Psychiatrist Interview

I have a feeling we pretty much adhered to our own concept of what we thought would be dangerous. I think we thought in terms of how likely is this man to do something very violent almost immediately after he's turned loose. And another criteria we used was "How would I feel having this man as my next-door neighbor?"

## Assumptions about the Need for Maximum Security

Patients who were deemed dangerous to themselves or others were those who were generally assumed to need maximum security. Although a decision about maximum security was technically a separate question, this decision usually followed the answer to the question about dangerousness. If one was dangerous, it was assumed that one needed to be in a maximum-security hospital. If one was not, it was assumed that one belonged in a less restrictive setting. The pairing of these assumptions are clear in the excerpt presented below.

Excerpt 6-21. From Final Evaluation Report of Team C

In conclusion, this is a delusion-ridden woman who is mentally ill [paranoid schizophrenia]. She is to be considered dangerous to others as she gives evidence of a hair-trigger temper and little compunction about violence. She is in need of a maximum-security setting and should, therefore, be retained at Lima State Hospital.

There were few exceptions to the assumption that dangerousness and need for maximum security go hand in hand. Two exceptions were systematically noted, however. The first involved a case where dangerousness was said to be unsure or unknown (a patient had only been in a hospital a short time). The second involved cases of "potentially" but not "immediately dangerous" patients who had a history of repeated escapes from civil mental hospitals. Althought the second type was observed as operative with only one team, both instances produced a recommendation of need for maximum security without ascription of dangerousness.

There were no general instances where patients were seen as immediately dangerous, but not recommended for maximum security. One example was noted wherein a team weighed its interviewing impression of dangerousness against a ten-year record of nonviolent institutional behavior. In that instance it was suggested that because of the patient's record of "good behavior," he merited a "trial prison stay." This was the exception to the rule, however, Present judgments of violence were ordinarily coordinated with past records of assault and future predictions of need for maximum security.

### Assumptions about "Psychopatic Offenders"

In considering patients committed under the inclusive Ascherman Act (Ohio's version of a sexual psychopath statute), team members were asked "to determine whether the individual is subject to continued commitment under recognized legal and medical standards."[8] The recognized standards with which teams were presented called for decisions as to whether an individual was mentally ill, mentally retarded, or a "psychopathic offender" and whether the patient continued to require the special custody and care provided by Lima State Hospital.[9]

I have already discussed assumptions about mental illness and retardation. This section focuses on assumptions about the psychopathic offender and the conditions which warrant continued custody and care. In actuality, most Ascherman patients are loosely categorized as psychopathic offenders. Hence, what we are really considering are the assumptions that team members made about patients confined within Lima State Hospital's special Ascherman Unit. Although some patients in this unit had never technically been classified as psychopathic offenders, it is evident from interviews with team members that the term "Ascherman" is generally equated with the terms "psychopath" or "sociopath."

Team members readily distinguished between mentally ill patients and Ascherman patients. Ascherman patients were repeatedly said not to be "psychotic" but were believed to possess that personality disorder referred to as either "psychopathy" or "sociopathy." Members were stereotypically uniform in making assumptions about "these kind" of patients as a whole. In interview after interview, and in observations of their discussions with each other, team members stated that the psychopathic offender was recognizable as an individual who had poor impulse control, a history of antisocial behavior, and was unable to learn from past experience. Moreover, such an individual was said to lack motivation, insight, the ability to enter into meaningful interpersonal relationships, and the ability to experience or show guilt. He or she was believed to be intelligent but without a moral sense or conscience, the master manipulator and con artist.

Excerpt 6-22. From Social Worker Interview

In the Ascherman Unit, of course, there was a big difference .... Ascherman people are not mentally ill. An Ascherman person is antisocial .... There's a big difference between a psychotic and a sociopath.

Excerpt 6-23. From Psychiatrist Interview

Ascherman patients [were] a group . . . without any mental aberration. OK, he has no mental illness. Here's an individual that acts out. This is a sociopath. It's a personality problem. And they're the con artists. You know, they're difficult ones to handle.
    Very few really change or benefit .... They repeat, repeat, repeat, repeat, repeat. Never learning from experience. This is why they carry the diagnosis. What we notice is that the histories [are] always pretty much broken homes, social problems background. And they start acting out and it became a problem, and then became a chronic problem. But they are the type of patient that either says, "Well, if I play along, why everything's going to be fine and I'll get out of here."

In approaching interviews with Ascherman patients, team members generally assumed that they themselves would become targets for manipulation. Because of this, some teams felt that they had to use special techniques, such as "stressing," to bring a sociopath's game to the surface.

Excerpt 6-24. From Social Worker Interview

I mean what can you say about a sociopath? . . . One of the things a sociopath will do—they're experts at manipulation and con games. They've lived their life this way, all their life. And, so they sure will—they'll try to manipulate you. . . . You have to use stress-manipulation. You have to use different kinds of techniques. A sociopath . . . you have to stress him.

Although they expected efforts to manipulate them, most teams did not feel that any special interview techniques were needed with psychopathic offenders. It was believed that simply asking them to relate the story of their offense and their feelings about violence would reveal whether or not these patients were trying to "con" team members into hearing things their way. As one clinician stated: "The Aschermans, they were going to convince us and tell us this is the way it is, and this is why they should be here, and this wasn't any good, and they're going to do this and all that." It was generally assumed that such "conning tactics" would become evident in the course of interviewing. Their answers would be "too right." They would have "excuses and explanations" for everything. Some members suggested that psychopathic patients probably practiced giving "acceptable responses." As one stated, "I think one thing they learned there [in the Ascherman Unit] was how to give the right answer at the right time." Another member commented that "at the Ascherman Unit they have these classes on how to interpret proverbs, which is ridiculous. I mean because they can't teach them that."

In the face of assumed manipulation, members appeared generally confident that they could sort out the real psychopathic offenders. Often this assumption appeared to open the door to a kind of circular reasoning by which any of a patient's statements might be taken as potentially manipulative. This circularity is revealed in the following excerpt. The interviewer is probing for any techniques that teams may have employed to sort out self-aggrandizing manipulative statements from honest statements, which nonetheless put a patient in a positive light.

Excerpt 6-25. From Psychiatrist Interview

*Interviewer*: How helpful were the patients' records in making your decisions?

*Psychiatrist*: I. Well, I found the records very helpful. . . . And I think, uh, particularly in the Ascherman Unit. I felt that the records really were essential. And, you know, as far as the sociopaths—to go in and interview them and expect to have some idea of whether they need to be there or not, you know, it's really, it'd be very egotistical.

*Interviewer*: That would be difficult. I guess part of the definition of the sociopath is that they try to manipulate you.

*Psychiatrist*: Uh humm.

*Interviewer*: Well, how did you deal with that during the interview? How did you discover whether an individual was trying to manipulate you? I mean, just saying things that a team might want to hear. I'm not sure how I'd do that: [pause], Was that a problem?

*Psychiatrist* [After a short pause]: Well, I think most, at least a lot of them, were [manipulative]. You mean in terms of what we did?

*Interviewer*: How would you be able to detect whether an individual was being manipulative? Was there any particular interview strategy that would give that impression? How would you tell if they were just being honest?

*Psychiatrist*: They just do it without any particular [laughs] . . . .

*Interviewer*: Oh, they just do it?

*Psychiatrist*: We didn't have to get them to manipulate. They just do it [laughs].

So far we have suggested that members generally assumed that Ascherman patients and psychopathic offenders were one and the same type of patient, that this type of patient possessed the various clinical traits associated with the diagnostic label psychopath or sociopath, and that this type of patient would ordinarily attempt to manipulate or "con" the review teams. In other areas the assumptions of members varied according to the teams in which they operated.

The first area in which team members' assumptions varied was that regarding recommendations for continued confinement and care. Once it was established that a patient fit the definition of a psychopathic offender, members made diverse assumptions as to whether or not a patient should stay in Lima special treatment units. The primary source of division was a contrast in assumptions about the treatability of psychopaths. Some teams appeared to operate on the assumption that treatment, particularly behavior modification,[10] could help a psychopathic offender to become more insightful, less manipulative, better able to handle interpersonal commitments, etc. These teams, like the law which mandates treatment prior to punishment,[11] assumed that real psychopaths were treatable. Hence, if in the process of diagnosing an individual it was concluded that he or she was psychopathic, it would be recommended that the patient still needed the confinement and care of Lima State's special unit. These teams (which believe in the treatability of psychopaths) also assumed that patients who were not clearly psychopaths (those who were already benefiting from treatment) should stay for more of the same. After all, it was reasoned, the kinds of programs from which patients were benefiting at Lima would not be available in the penal settings in which patients were liable to be placed. Thus, the only patients for whom continued care was not assumed to be needed were those "nonpsychopathic" individuals who had nothing more to learn from the treatment available at Lima.

Other teams clearly assumed that real psychopathic offenders could not benefit from treatment. Once these teams established that a patient was typically psychopathic, they routinely recommended that he or she no longer needed the special care and confinement of Lima State Hospital. This assumption is displayed in the following discussion of one review team.

Excerpt 6-26. From Patient Review 430, Team B

(461) *Psychiatrist*: Why don't we say it like we feel it, then? Why don't we say that this guy has not improved. He's not recovered. He's not mentally ill. I'm sorry, he's not psychotic. He's not retarded. He is mentally ill. He's a psychopathic offender. But we can see nothing to be gained by his continued hospitalization here, and there isn't any reason why he can't or should not be returned to jail.

(462) *Psychologist*: And even though he has not recovered it doesn't look like he's going to benefit from treatment. . . .

(463) *Psychiatrist*: Yes, yeah. How about that?

The assumption of "nontreatability" is modified by several correlative assumptions. The first suggests that the inability to treat psychopathy decreases with the increased age of the individual. In effect, this proposition assumes that psychopathy must be "outgrown" or "burnt-out." Note the operative use of this idea in the following excerpts.

Excerpt 6-27. From Patient Review 440, Team D

(485)  *Social Worker*: You're not saying he'll never feel like changing, 'cuz you can't say never. . . .

(486)  *Psychiatrist*: I'm only saying that at age forty, forty-five, fifty, he'll maybe be in the clink again, but, uh, he may be somewhat adjusting to society on the basis of age only, not on the basis of any particular kind of program. 'Cuz the psychopathy in a sense, tends to fade after let's say thirty-five or forty.

Two other modifiers to the assumption about nontreatability were observed. The first occurred in cases where, although a psychopathic patient did not appear to be learning greater insight through treatment, it was felt that his or her behavior had become more restrained or controlled by being in Lima. In such situations it was generally felt that the benefits of control were such to merit a statement that the patient continued to need the special custody offered by the Ascherman Unit. The second modifier concerned psychopathic patients who had spent only a short time (usually less than a year) in the special Ascherman Unit. One team, in particular, used this "time spent at Lima" variable as a regular index for whether or not a nontreatable patient should continue to be confined in the special unit. Although this team never expressed confidence in the efficacy of such treatment, it appeared to operate on the assumption that since a treatment setting was available, eligible patients might as well spend some time there.

With the exception of the modifiers discussed above, teams which assumed the nontreatability of the psychopathic offender recommended that such patients be released from Lima. This recommendation carried with it no sense that the patient was progressing or that he or she was cured. Actually it was often made because teams believed that penal settings were the most appropriate places for controlling the behaviors of the "untreatable" social deviants.

Excerpt 6-28. From Patient Review 443, Team D

(534)  *Social Worker*: Well, why not send him to prison? What's he going to get out of being here?

(535)  *Psychiatrist*: Well, you could say that he doesn't necessarily need to be here.

(536)  *Social Worker*: That's what I'm saying.

(537)  *Psychiatrist*: Oh, oh, all right. No problem. He just requires the care and custody of a respective training institution is all. . . .

(538)   *Social Worker*: Yeah, that's why I related it to the other case. He said he isn't in here. . . .

(539)   *Psychiatrist*: Oh yeah. I see what you mean. I was just talking about the fact of incarceration, not of whether he needs Lima specifically.

Of the five teams for which we had most data regarding decisions about psychopathic offenders, teams L and G made the assumption of treatability, while teams B, D, and J assumed that treatment did not help. Within the "nontreatability" grouping, however, there was no consensus as to what to do with patients who were benefiting from treatment (who were not truly psychopaths). Team B tended to recommend continued care for patients in this category, but teams D and J did not. This difference is accounted for in teams of other assumptions that these teams made about the helpfulness of the Lima program itself. Team B believed that what "improving" (nonpsychopathic) patients could get out of the Ascherman Unit was better than what they'd get in prison. Teams D and J, on the other hand, appeared to believe that "relatively well" patients would benefit more by returning to a penal setting, where they had more freedom and stood a chance of being paroled earlier and thus returning to the community. These differential assumptions are displayed below.

Excerpt 6-29. From Patient Review 421, Team B

(152)   *Psychologist*: That's my only concern, that I think there's something treatable there. And it would be a crime to miss it. He's not going to get it at Chillicothe and I don't think he's going to get it at any of the penitentiaries.

Excerpt 6-30. From Patient Review 441, Team D

(In this excerpt Team D expresses its understanding of the legal advantages of getting "relatively well" patients out of Lima.)

(420)   *Psychiatrist*: He doesn't need the maximum care and custody of this, but that doesn't say that we might be condemning him to some place worse. If some of the tales. . . .

(421)   *Psychologist*: Yeah, right. If he's to ever get out, he's got to get out of here first.

(422)   *Psychiatrist*: Right. I guess.

(423)   *Psychologist*: Now that I know, because they won't release you directly from here, with his term.

Excerpt 6-31. From Patient Review 440, Team D

(This excerpt documents Team D's assumption that things are "freer" and "more open" for patient prisoners in a correctional setting.)

(566)   *Social Worker*: This is much more confining here than other penal institutions. A number of the patients are trying to get out of here and go to the prison. There's much more freedom. You can walk around.

A second area of general difference in assumptions about psychopathic offenders focused on what teams believed "they had to say" about a patient who was to need further custody. Teams differed as to whether they had to label an individual as a "psychopathic offender" if they recommended continued confinement. This assumptive difference followed the manner in which teams interpreted restraints placed upon their work by the laws and the court order. Some teams believed that only "psychopathic offenders" could stay in the special unit. Hence, if a patient was felt not to be a psychopathic offender, but was benefiting from the treatment offered by the unit, the patient was called a psychopathic offender anyway. Although this was done in the interest of the patients, the diagnostic label "psychopathic offender" was entered into the patient's permanent record, even though the label was believed to be clinically incorrect.

Teams which assumed that it was necessary to mislabel patients as "psychopathic offenders" in order to procure treatment appeared to resolve potential dissonance by suggesting that the patient was "legally" if not "psychiatrically" a psychopathic offender. In the long run, however, they may have endangered the patient's future options by affixing a label that could be relied upon by future diagnosticians. The operation of this assumption is revealed in the subsequent excerpts.

Excerpt 6-32. From Patient Review 421, Team B

(115) *Psychiatrist*: There's one bit of reality we have to face, that if we call him a psychopathic offender. . . .

(116) *Psychologist*: All right, but I'm—when I said he didn't seem to be a sociopath, I'm going along with the idea that he's a sociopathic offender, uh. . . . This guy, by the time he's thirty, might be mentally ill, therefore, diagnose the whole, that potential kind of thing. I'm saying this guy might. . . . He needs to be somewhere for a while. It's not going to be short-term therapy. Put him out on the street now and he's going to be back in trouble again. He's simply more of an inadequate personality than an antisocial personality.

(117) *Psychiatrist*: Well, he's antisocial by action.

(118) *Psychologist*: Yeah, behaviorally he's. . . . Antisocial personality is a psychiatric label and I can't go along with that.

(119) *Social Worker*: Well, then you're saying that if he stays you don't mind seeing him as a psychopathic offender, and having treatment.

The psychologist in the interaction presented above later makes explicit what the social worker is suggesting. He concludes that "in order to keep him here we'd have to label him a psychopathic offender." Other teams do not assume such to be the case. They tend to affix a less powerful clinical label (that is, "inadequate personality") to patients who they recommend for further treatment. Note, for instance, the denial of any need to call "nonpsychopaths" something which they are not, as it is depicted in the following excerpt:

Excerpt 6-33. From Patient Review 441, Team D

(411)    *Psychiatrist*: We have split here. Well, is he a psychopathic offender? In the psychiatric-psychological sense [this] is a little different than [*sic*] it is in the legal sense.

(412)    *Social Worker*: Yeah.

(413)    *Psychiatrist*: And that's all we're talking about. Sure the law has to do what it says it has to do, but this guy is not helpless. He does have some insights. He has some expectations. And he has a fifty-fifty chance of maybe getting probation. I think there's a drive toward, uh—how do I say. . . .

(414)    *Psychologist*: There's less.

(415)    *Psychiatrist*: Yeah. Less antisocial kinds of behavior.

(416)    *Psychologist*: Right.

(417)    *Psychiatrist*: I think we could simply avoid the psychopathic offender bit and not even say he's recovered or not.

So far we have discussed varying assumptions about whether teams had to use the label "psychopathic offender" if they wanted a patient to stay. A similar question arose for teams who wanted a particular patient to leave. Could they call him a "psychopathic offender" anyway? Some teams believed that they could, as long as they prefaced their diagnostic remarks with statements suggesting that the patient had nothing more to gain from treatment (assuming that a psychopathic offender was not treatable). Others felt that they had better not affix the label "psychopathic offender" because then the patient would inevitably stay at Lima. Such an assumption is displayed below:

Excerpt 6-34. From Patient Review 443, Team D

(The team is beginning to formulate their final report. They have already decided the patient should be transferred.)

(526)    *Social Worker*: Mr. 433 is a psychopathic offender. . . .

(527)    *Psychologist*: Oh, wait a minute. If we say that, he stays here.

(528)    *Psychiatrist*: Right [pause].

(529)    *Social Worker*: Well, you know I don't want to say that, but that's what he is.

The team in the above excerpt didn't want the patient to stay, yet they thought he should be classified as a "psychopathic offender." But if they classified him as they thought he should be properly classified, they believed that he would have to stay. Rather than saying he was "not a psychopathic offender" and committing themselves to a diagnosis which they believed to be incorrect,

119

they decided to skirt the whole issue. They would simply say nothing about the psychopathic offender issue and speak only to the question regarding need for continued custody and care. The consequences of this, however, would be that a patient who was felt to be "psychopathic" would not be referred to as such in the team's entry on his permanent record.

Excerpt 6–35. From Patient Review 443, Team D

(589)   *Social Worker*: You're not going to call him a psychopathic offender?

(590)   *Psychologist*: No. He is, but. . . .

(591)   *Psychiatrist*: We don't have to diagnose him.

(592)   *Psychologist*: No, they want us to tell, they want us to tell them whether or not. . . .

(593)   *Psychiatrist*: He needs to be here.

(594)   *Psychologist*: Yes or no.

(595)   *Social Worker*: Mr. [443] no longer needs the special custody, care, or treatment provided by Lima State Hospital.

In reviewing members' assumptions about the psychopathic offender, we have seen that in several areas assumptions appear to be very similar. In other areas, such as those related to beliefs about treatability and the need to label retained patients "psychopathic offenders," teams are quite split. We have seen, moreover, that differences in assumptions often produce differences in patients' recommended fates. This leads us to conclude that the ways that teams differentially frame such clinical assumptions are important determinants of what are presented to the court as final diagnostic decisions.

*Concluding Remarks*

In the preceding pages we have considered two types of framings: those that structure members' purposes-at-hand and those organizing assumptions about relevant clinical-legal categories. These framings serve to delimit or focus the substance and form of final diagnostic decisions. Nonetheless, the framing of purposes and assumptions operates only within an ongoing process of social interaction. That is, they become only more or less relevant, more or less operative, depending on the situated perceptions, needs, and judgment of members at a given point in social time and space. In the following three chapters, I shall address the issue of these situated interactional processes. In the next chapter, we shall attempt to understand them in terms of members' work in previewing patients by surveying an individuals past record.

**Notes**

1. The multi-focused aspect of human interaction is also suggested by Goffman. In *Frame Analysis* he implies that the consideration of human experience as framed by one definition of the situation is more an analytical construction than an existential description.

2. A minor distinction should be made between what the court technically ordered and what teams practically did or "overdid." For those ruled not guilty by reason of insanity, the court technically called for a decision about mental illness or retardation and dangerousness, but not maximum security per se. For penal transfers, the court ordered judgments about mental illness or retardation and maximum security, but not dangerousness. In practice teams tended to make statements about all three assessment categories for both classifications of patients. In other words, addressing either the dangerousness or maximum-security issue seemed to imply addressing the other issue as well.

3. This issue will be considered further in our discussion of assumptions regarding "psychopathy." Yet, it is important to note that many members referred to Ascherman patients (those hospitalized as psychopathic offenders) as really the most dangerous of patients.

4. The assumption that psychiatric professionals are better able to predict who won't be dangerous than who will be dangerous is supported by recent research. Cf. H.R. Kozol, R. Boucher, and R. Garofalo, "The Diagnosis and Treatment of Dangerousness," *Crime and Delinquency* 18 (October 1972): 371-392.

5. Note the reliance on the past record of assaultiveness in this final report of Team L.

Excerpt from Final Evaluation Report of Team L

The chart indicates that his stay at this institution [for two years] has been without incident and he has been maintained on medication adequately.... [During the interview] the patient was in good contact with reality, friendly, in no acute distress and showing no evidence of memory impairment. He verbalized good intentions for the future and a strong desire to return to society.

In spite of his apparent stabilized condition at this time, it is the feeling of this review group that in view of his chronic schizophrenic condition, in view of his lengthy history of acting out behavior, dangerously so at times, we feel this patient is dangerous and continues to be.

6. Teams occasionally, questioned the adequacy of incident reports that were filed in a patient's record. As one psychologist observed: "Sometimes our team found that a patient was put in seclusion for not doing something an attendant wanted him to do, but the patient never physically acted out." In the following excerpt we find another team member suggesting that the records may underreport violence as well.

Excerpt from Social Worker Interview

In a lot of cases there was very little to document that a guy was dangerous. Now, he may have been much more dangerous than what was in the record. In a few cases we found, for example, a newspaper clipping, which kind of clarified why the guy was at Lima State. In those cases you had a piece of journalism which in some ways informed you a lot better than the admission record or the psychiatric history.

7. The situational character of violence is recognized by the psychologist in the following excerpt.

Excerpt from Interview with Psychologist

The phrase "extreme likelihood of immediate danger" was a tough point because it was a situational diagnosis. We look in the folder . . . at a patient's past record and how he had been dangerous before [and at] what he had done during his period of incarceration. [But] we had to work through all sorts of situational dynamics [including] the medication and the patient's reaction on and off it.

8. For a detailed discussion of the Ascherman Act (Section 2945.25 of the Ohio Revised Code) see James M. Caulfield, "Ohio Commitments of the Mentally Ill Offender," *Capital University Law Review* 4, 1 (1974): 27-35.

9. These standards were borrowed from the wording of the Ascherman Act in the Ohio Revised Code 2947.25 (G). They were presented and explained to team members by representatives of the Ohio Division of Mental Health and its Office of Forensic Psychiatry.

10. In this regard it is important to note that the treatment program in Lima's special "Ascherman Unit" was an intermingling of behavior modification and patient self-government approaches to therapy.

11. The fact that "cured" patients facing the prospect of having their sentences reinstated so that they could receive the proper punishment of the penal system is one of the inherent contradictions of the so-called Ascherman Act.

# 7 Previewing the Diagnostic Work: Preinterview Discussion by Review Team Members

*[The patient's case record] is apparently not used to record occasions when the patient showed capacity to cope honorably and effectively with difficult situations. Nor is the case record typically used to provide a rough average or sampling of his past conduct. [Rather, it extracts] from his whole life course a list of those incidents that have or might have had "symptomatic" significance. . . . I think most of the information is quite true, although it might seem also to be true that almost anyone's life course could yield up enough denigrating facts to provide grounds for the record's justification of commitment.*

> Erving Goffman, *Asylums* (Chicago: Aldine, 1962), pp. 155, 159

Before interviewing patients, review team members engaged in two kinds of "pre-viewing." They preview the decision-making tasks required by this "type" of patient. They preview the patient through a consideration of his or her past record. In this chapter we examine each of these previewings. Together these represent the first step in the social construction of patients' psychiatric realities.

## Previewing the Task

Teams routinely use their preinterview discussions about a particular case to negotiate and display their assumptions about types or categories of patients and what it is that they must determine for each. This occurs most frequently when teams receive the record of a patient belonging to some category with which they have not yet worked (psychopathic offender, penal transfer, etc.).

Previewing the formal task often involves both an instrumental and evaluative component. Instrumentally, teams display knowledge of what they are supposed to decide for patients in a certain category. Evaluatively, teams comment on what they feel about either the required decision or the patients within a particular category. Both of these components are revealed in the following excerpt. The team involved is about to review its first Ascherman ("psychopathic offender") case.

124

Excerpt 7-1. From Patient Review 430, Team B

(9) *Psychiatrist*: Let's uh . . . do you want to review the Ascherman thing first?

(10) *Psychologist*: Yeah, that's what I'm looking at here.

(11) *Psychiatrist*: For us?

(12) *Psychologist*: Supposedly they have to be seen within 120 days from the commencement of the evaluation procedures.

(13) *Psychiatrist*: All right.

(14) *Psychologist*: [reads section of the interim court order outlining require-ments for reviewing Ascherman cases. The psychologist concludes with the following remark]: So what we need to decide is whether or not these people have improved to the point that they no longer need. . . .

(15) *Social Worker*: The special custody.

(16) *Psychologist*: Right. Which essentially means they'll either be probated or they'll be sentenced. This is all presentencing.

(17) *Hospital Security Guard*: [poking his head into the small conference room]: Excuse me. We have [the patient's name] on this ward.

(18) *Psychologist*: Alrighty. [The guard leaves again.] So that is what the Ascherman is, presentencing, and our decision is whether or not he needs to be here. If he doesn't then we can assume that he either goes back to court for sentencing or he's freed.

(19) *Psychiatrist*: Which is kind of scary.

(20) *Psychologist*: Did you say kind of scary?

(21) *Psychiatrist*: Well, these are a bunch of scary boys we've got today.

(22) *Social Worker*: Are they?

(23) *Psychologist*: These aren't the easy ones, huh, [psychiatrist's name]?

(24) *Psychiatrist*: No.

(25) *Social Worker*: Saving the best till last.

In the preceding excerpt, one notes a clear differentiation between the instru-mental assertions in lines (9) through (12) and the evaluative commentary in lines (19) through (25). In characterizing Ascherman patients as a "scary bunch of boys," the team is developing a theme which it will repeatedly use as an index of patients who "really" belong to this category in its subsequent decision-making. Other teams display evaluative typings that are more positive. In the following excerpt, for instance, a simple observation that a particular patient will be having visitors leads to the display of assumed knowledge about the better psychiatric condition of Ascherman patients as a whole.

Excerpt 7-2. From Patient Review 442, Team D

(47) *Psychologist*: [referring to patients gathered for interviews by a hospital security guard]: He got them for me already, quick worker. That's funny, they said [patient 442] is out for a visit. Does that mean he's out front?

(48) *Psychiatrist*: Yeah, his relatives are visiting.

(49) *Psychologist*: Oh, OK. I thought maybe they had a trial leave or something, because it says here [in the records] "escapee." [All laugh. Members then digress in a short discussion of the patient's medication history and date of admission. After this the team pauses and the social worker reintroduces the discussion about having visitors.]

(69) *Social Worker*: I wonder why they don't use a bigger room for visiting than the place down front.

(70) *Psychologist*: Apparently people are visiting up here [on the ward], too.

(71) *Social Worker*: Oh, are they? No kidding?

(72) *Psychiatrist*: Yeah, they use every available space.

(73) *Social Worker*: I didn't think they let anybody through the building.

(74) *Psychiatrist*: Well, maybe when they design a building, they don't count on crowds of visitors.

(75) *Social Worker*: It's interesting this group [Ascherman patients] has more visitors per capita than any we've seen in the main building.

(76) *Psychologist*: Oh, yeah.

(77) *Psychiatrist*: Well, they're probably younger so there's a few people still around to visit them and uh. . . .

(78) *Social Worker*: But then there's also the fact that they're sane, whereas in the other building they're out of their heads. People feel there's no use. You can't talk to them, no relationship.

Often teams' previewing of their tasks was concerned less with distinctions about patients than it was with the relationship between their work and the work of the legal sector, the constraints of the court order, or the criminal code. Teams generally thematized this relationship so that the legal sector was viewed as concerned with "adjudicating" a patient's fate, while evaluation teams were seen as "discovering" what a patient was really like. The legal sector was seen as the real decision-makers. The psychiatric sector (the review teams themselves) was seen as simply professional diagnosticians. In the following excerpt, we find a team displaying this distinction between the "adjudicative mission" of the court and the "discovery mission" of the patient reviewers. The team is discussing their task in reviewing Ascherman patients.

126

Excerpt 7-3. From Patient Review 420, Team B

(29)  *Psychologist*: Are we supposed to go for that label or not? Say whether or not they are now psychopathic offenders?

(30)  *Psychiatrist*: I guess so.

(31)  *Psychologist*: For each one received today?

(32)  *Psychiatrist*: Yes. We're supposed to say whether they're improved or recovered.

(33)  *Social Worker*: Its almost a foregoing thing.

(34)  *Psychiatrist*: Its almost pointless to say that.

(35)  *Psychologist*: If they're a psychopathic offender they're going to stay here?

(36)  *Psychiatrist*: Yes.

(37)  *Psychologist*: [referring to the patient whose record is being considered]: This guy's been labeled an "antisocial personality."

(38)  *Social Worker*: He [referring to the psychiatrist] said they're all going back to court anyway.

(39)  *Psychologist*: All of these people whether we label them psychopathic offender or not are going back to court anyway?

(40)  *Psychiatrist*: Yes.

(41)  *Social Worker*: They're all going back?

(42)  *Psychologist*: What's the difference. . . . Here's a man labeled psychopathic offender and he goes back to court, and a man we say is not a psychopathic offender—he goes back to court too? Then what?

(43)  *Psychiatrist*: It's not for us to determine where they go.

(44)  *Psychologist*: That's right. The court takes the final ruling—whether he stays here, goes to jail, et cetera.

The team above has concluded that the court is the real adjudicator of where patients go. This typical conclusion pays little attention to the fact that the court relies almost exclusively on the opinion of the psychiatric teams in its decisions. Nor does it account for the fact that teams (including that excerpted) routinely couch their diagnostic wordings so that they secure the legal outcomes which are believed to be psychiatrically most appropriate. (We have already touched on this matter in our previous discussion of differential assumptions related to the diagnosis of the psychopathic offender.) In not thematizing these matters, members appear to promote images of their "expert identities." As experts, their task is discovery. They should stay clear of the mundane legal entanglements that are the domain of the court and the criminal code. These issues are summarized in the instructive monologue of a psychiatrist in the following excerpt. Reviewers are told that they "shouldn't worry too much about the [legal] code" and that they shouldn't lose sight of their expert mission as "behavioral scientists."

Excerpt 7-4. From Patient Review 40, Team G

(The psychiatrist is responding to a question to what statutory category a patient falls under. He begins his rather lengthy remarks by stating: "I think we shouldn't worry too much about the code." The following is excerpted from the last section of his "monologue.")

So our determination is to find whether he's retarded or insane, or whether he's dangerous, and then we can talk about him. Any questions about? Do you have any...? The point I'm making is if we get, we can't get hung up in those codes. Because if we do, we uh, we're like lawyers. We lose sight of what we're here for as behavioral scientists, you know. We can always contest the code later on . . . in what our finding in our report is.

It is interesting to note that while the team is instructed to disregard the code, they are simultaneously reminded that they can "contest the code" in their formulation of a final report. Hence, they can both project an image as disinterested professional "discoverers" and, at the same time, exert power in controlling the actual direction of judicial decisions. This is a major theme, interwoven in many of the review team discussions. Like the thematizations of assumptions about patients, it is often displayed in the preinterview conversations of members.

## Previewing the Patient through the Record

The importance of the past record for members' "discoveries" about patients cannot be overstated. Most teams used information from the past record to formulate and display "theories" about patients' present psychiatric status. Of nine teams observed reviewing the record before interviewing patients, seven consistently used the record to construct present images of the patient. The two teams evidencing "less theorizing" still occasionally revealed "summary judgments" about patients from readings of past clinical notes and entries.[1] The kind of preinterviewing theorizing with which I am concerned is clearly displayed in the following excerpt.

Excerpt 7-5. From Patient Review 422, Team B

(2) *Psychiatrist*: Escapee . . . [patient's name]. . . . You know what that means; I'll tell you what that means. It means that sometime in the past, maybe in jail, maybe ten years ago, a guy escaped and they're required to put Escapee on their chart, it doesn't mean anything at all. I have very little on him, too. He's a

nineteen-year-old . . . oh . . . I know he's the nineteen-year-old kid who got busted and who got a twenty-to-forty-year sentence for selling acid.

(3)    *Psychologist*: Sounds like New York state.

(4)    *Social Worker*: I was going to say it looks justified. . . .

(5)    *Psychiatrist*: But he has a long history. . . .

(6)    *Social Worker*: He's not a nice kid. . . .

(7)    *Psychiatrist*: He's been a drug user, a drug pusher. They don't like this. They say all his life he's lied, he's stolen, he's exhibited no moral sense.

(8)    *Social Worker*: [reading from record]: Cruel to animals, set fire to the neighbors. . . .

(9)    *Psychiatrist*: Breaking and entering, auto theft. . . .

(10)    *Social Worker*: . . . Never loyal to anyone, no moral sense of people.

(11)    *Psychologist*: There was an old study in terms of violence, too, and we haven't even discussed this, but, if a kid before the age of, whatever, ten, has been cruel to animals, had a problem with setting of fires, and suffered any . . ., there was like a 90 percent chance of violent. . . .

(12)    *Psychiatrist*: He's been to JDC, BYS. IQ of 109.

(13)    *Psychologist*: Yep.

(14)    *Psychiatrist*: He's never really worked. He's doing very well in the hospital.

(15)    *Psychologist*: It sounds like we do have a stone here.

(16)    *Psychiatrist*: We have what?

(17)    *Psychologist*: Stone.

(18)    *Psychiatrist*: Is that the term for the . . . ?

(19)    *Psychologist*: No, that's our little private term, stone-cold psychopath.

(20)    *Psychiatrist*: Yeah.

(21)    *Psychologist*: That last guy we saw I don't think was. I wouldn't classify him Stone.

(22)    *Psychiatrist*: He's not stone cold.

(23)    *Psychologist*: Right. When he's on the street, he acts pretty stone cold, I bet. But it's situational. If you could work with it, while it's here. He's not adapting as well as the other guys. He'll get the hang of it. [This statement was in reference to the previous patient. The psychologist now continues to discuss the patient at hand.] What about relationships? Wife, girl friend, mother, father?

(24)    *Psychiatrist*: He is single. I think he talks about getting a raw deal. . . .

(25)    *Psychologist*: Oh, yeah. . . .

(26)    *Psychologist*: A wooden leg! [This statement is in reference to an item

the social worker has noted in the patient's chart.] I can't help it. "Look at me, I've got a wooden leg."

(27) *Psychiatrist*: Talk about rationalization. Wait till we get downstairs. They're loaded.

(28) *Social Worker*: Oh, really?

(35) *Psychiatrist*: His parents are divorced and he never got along with his stepfather.

(36) *Psychologist*: What about the mother? This guy probably never got along with anybody.

(37) *Social Worker*: Right [reading from chart]. He's self-centered and doesn't want to take the time to get help. . . .

(38) *Psychologist*: That's 'cause nothing ever bothered him [pause].

From the very first line, the team uses the materials in the past record to make theoretical inferences about the patient in the present. This is a clear example of the process of documentary interpretation. The appearance of the patient (through second-hand reports inscribed in the record) are taken as documents of an invariant underlying pattern. The "escapee" designation, drug arrests, and long history (line 2), not only look justified (line 4), but show that "he's not a nice kid" (line 6). The appearance of a list of particular behaviors (cruelty to animals, setting fire, breaking and entering, etc.) are viewed as indicators that he is a particular kind of person. He is someone who is "never loyal to anyone" and has no moral sense of people (line 10).

In line (11), the emergent theorizing about the patient is legitimated by fitting him into a stock of typified clinical knowledge about persons who have similar characteristics. This reference to the findings of "an old study" expands the team's cognitive grasp of what the patient is really like. In all likelihood, the patient is a violent type person as well.

In lines (14) to (20), this interpretation is complete. This "not nice kid" never really worked, yet "he's doing well in the hospital" (line 14). Perhaps his "success" is due to his manipulation of appearances. Clearly, this is what is implied by the psychologist's statement: "It sounds like we do have a stone here" (line 15). The psychiatric essence of the patient is his psychopathic personality.

The interpretation of the patient as a "stone-cold psychopath" is supported by certain indexical resources available to team members in their particular diagnostic setting. One such contextual resource is cognitive. Team members are able to situationally employ stocks of clinical knowledge to display the reasonableness of a present interpretation in light of "past findings." The situated citation of the results of "an old study" (line 11) is an example of such cognitive indexicality.

The comparison of the present patient with "the last guy we saw" (line 21) is also an example of the indexical nature of the interpretive process. Here the indexicality is rooted in the concreteness of recently lived experience rather than in the situated use of past abstractions.[2] The result, however, is the same—the contextual generation of knowledge; the situational transformation of observed "appearances" into known "facts" (or invariant essences). The previous guy wasn't a "stone." It was "situational" with him. But with "this guy" it is different. He not only appears to be a stone, he is a stone.

Once the deviant identity of the patient is known as a "stone-cold psychopath," other aspects of the record are "reflexively" seen as additional supports to this conclusion. "He is single" and "I think he talks about getting a raw deal" (line 24) are given a new clinical meaning. Being single, especially for a nineteen-year-old, could mean or not mean almost anything. In the context of viewing a psychopath, however, it assumes the reflexive significance of representing additional evidence. After all, it is believed that such individuals cannot form meaningful relationships. Likewise, "talking about getting a raw deal" can be reflexively viewed as "rationalizing," another sign of psychopathy. The psychiatrist's response—"Oh, yeah" in line (25)—is indicative that such is the way these statements were heard.

After the process of reflexively "reading into" the record is begun, it seems to snowball. In line (26), the psychologist mimics what is supposed to be the patient's manipulative rationalization connected with having a wooden leg. Under other circumstances, the fact of such a physical impairment may have engendered sympathy. For a "known" psychopath, however, this is just an additional bit of data by which to recognize the kind of person the patient "really" is. "Talk about rationalizations" responds the psychiatrist (line 27), indicating that he concurs with the psychologist's inferences. These are extended by categorization of this patient as the same type as those found in the ward "downstairs" where "they're loaded [with psychopaths]."

Lines (35) and (36) are complements of lines (24) to (25) and (26) to (27). In the previous pairings, the psychologist cites data suggestive of a reading of the patient as a psychopath. The responses of the psychiatrist ("Oh, yeah" and "Talk about rationalizations") provide collaborative confirmation of these reflexive inferences. In line (35), the psychiatrist presents additional inferential materials. ("His parents are divorced and he never got along with his stepfather.") In line (36), the psychologist confirms the psychiatrist's inference through answering his own question. "What about the mother? This guy probably never got along with anybody.")

In a short series of exchanges about a few items in the record, the team has apparently figured the patient out. They have come to a theoretical understanding of the kind of person he is in the present through an indexical and reflexive reading of other persons' statements about his past. The treating of "past statements" as "present seeings" is nowhere clearer than in line (37). "Right," begins the social worker, concurring with the previous observation that the patient "probably never got along with anybody." "He's self-centered and doesn't want to take the time to get help." The psychologist confirms this reading and gives closure to the team's prejudgment of the patient by commenting, "That's 'cause nothing ever bothered him." The basis for this "expert insight" is apparently the reflexive build-up of a particular image of the patient in the preceding exchanges.

The preinterview theorizing about patients is extremely important because it determines or selectively focuses members' expectations about who it is they are going to interview. This channeling of expectations is revealed in case after case.

### Excerpt 7-6. From Patient Review 71, Team J

(The observer has approached the team about having patients sign the necessary research consent form. The psychiatrist's comments concern whether or not "this type" of patient will give the consent.)

(11) *Research Observer*: Uh, they should, I guess, uh, maybe we should ask them if they could sign it.

(12) *Psychiatrist*: Yeah, when they come in. I was going to say this [name of patient 71], he's really a kind of a paranoid black activist. It will be interesting. Well, we'll see what he says. I think he will [sign the consent form]. We'll just explain it's nothing to do with him, but the way we're conducting the interviews and evaluations.

### Excerpt 7-7. From Patient Review 421, Team B

(In this series of exchanges, the team used the patient's "age" as a previewing index of his likely psychopathy.)

(26) *Psychiatrist*: Well, I hate to admit this but my mind is made up on these people even before we see them.

(27) *Psychologist*: Well, there is, uh.... We do have to.... It's a matter of degree here.

(28) *Social Worker*: It's a matter of degree in terms of whether they stay here now or go back to court right away.

(29) *Psychiatrist*: Yeah. Well, I'll admit I'm a little prejudiced but I'm going to withhold my judgment. Basically what this guy is, what, twenty-two years of age. It's not just that he's into it. He's a psychopathic offender and he should stay here a longer time.... Well, I don't know....

(31-35) (Team digresses for a few exchanges on whether all patients go immediately back to court. The psychologist then reintroduces the "theorizing" about the meaning of the patient's age.)

(36) *Psychologist*: Twenty-two is just a bad age to be working on these guys.

(37) *Social Worker*: Yeah. They haven't learned.

(38) *Psychologist*: The twenties is the worst decade to be a psychopath....

(39) *Psychiatrist*: They haven't burned out yet.

Excerpt 7-8. From Patient Review 361, Team L

(The psychiatrist completes his review of the record with the following summary judgment.)

(15) *Psychiatrist*: He had a cocky attitude but does not cause any major difficulties to the program or its function. He's workable for therapy, but will need an extended period of time to achieve the necessary insight and emotional maturation. This case will be reevaluated later. So in other words, we already have the answer—that he still needs treatment.

(16) *Psychologist*: Clearly true.

Excerpt 7-9. From Patient Review 112, Team A

(The team is reviewing the record of patient found previously to be "incompetent to stand trial.")

(41) *Psychiatrist*: Well, this is what I mean. This guy is not dumb. He's the type who probably really knew what was going on. So he cops an insanity plea just to get off the hook.

In each preceding excerpt, summary judgments from the record are used to shape an image of a patient yet to be interviewed, whether teams alert themselves to such things as the "paranoia of a black activist" (excerpt 7-7), the ability to be treated because of "no major difficulties in the program" (excerpt 7-8), and likely malingering due to "not being dumb" (excerpt 7-9). Theorizing from the previewed past casts shadows on what the patient is imagined to be in the present. It creates a perceptual set with which teams approach patients. Patients labeled as extremely dangerous, for instance, were often approached by teams with considerable apprehension.

Excerpt 7-10. From Psychiatrist Interview

In terms of dangerousness we would check the past record. This gave us a pretty good idea about past performance. And when it showed considerable acting out, it was that we were generally not fearful but apprehensive, to say the least, as to their possibility of striking out right there and then.

Although preinterview theorizing was a common practice of most review teams, the particular way in which this previewing was done was not always agreed upon. Occasionally, disagreement arose as to the most adequate theoretical framework through which to preconceive patients. One such disagreement is displayed below. Yet, even in disagreeing about the documents for a particular interpretation, both parties still assume that present knowledge can be indexically constructed from past representations.

Excerpt 7-11. From Patient Review 365, Team L

(8)  *Psychologist*: He's a remarkable guy who was the product of many years of bad family but has managed to learn something from it.

(9)  *Social Worker*: You know what he sounds like to me? You know, in a prison structure there is always the bit con that controls or appears [to be] the saint of thing, but behind he has got little henchman.

(10)  *Psychologist*: Absolutely wrong picture here. We're dealing with the people who are not in the same prison setting. Yes, in a prison setting you do have those guys who rise up to the top. But in the world of the psychopath he comes across as a guy with insights, sincerity, and some ability to change. And that's why I think he's very, very different from the person you described.

The two members in the previous excerpt are not in disagreement over interpreting the patient's present through documents of his past. Their disagreement is concerned with the "indexical" particulars which most appropriately reveal the essence of the patient's personality. The social worker (indexically) contextualizes the patient against the background of "incarcerated convicts." The psychologist selects a population of "hospitalized psychopaths" as a point of (indexical) reference. The product of each interpretive framework is obviously different. The social worker, however, does not accept the psychologist's redefinition of the situation. Throughout the patient interview, the social worker pursues a line of questioning related to the "big con" theory. The psychologist, on the other hand, asked questions directed at documenting the "he's a remarkable guy" thesis. These divergent perspectives await the negotiations of the postinterview discussion. Yet, despite difference, these interpretations are representative of the manner in which preinterview theorizing selectively focused attention to particular aspects of a patient's psychiatric reality.

Instances in which members actually questioned the merits of preinterview theorizing were quite rare. This practice was ordinarily taken for granted. On occasion, however, particular team members were observed "calling into question" or placing boundaries around the extensive use of such previewing. In the following excerpt a psychiatrist reminds members that there is a difference between theory and fact. This reminder is noteworthy because of its relative uncommonness.

Excerpt 7-12. From Patient Review 443, Team D

(The psychologist and social worker are here collaborating in the construction of particular psychiatric identity for a patient prior to the actual interview. The "data" they employ is drawn solely from the past record.)

(118)  *Social Worker*: Well, it fits with the picture of poor relationship with the father. Authority figures—rebelliousness against authority, social fears.

(119)  *Psychologist*: Fears of inferiority.

(120)   *Social Worker*: Feelings of inadequacy, incompetent, not. . . . He's really getting some fun out of this, too. There also could be a problem of marital relationship.

(121)   *Psychiatrist*: Well, it is indicated in there that he likes to have it every-day and his wife would only give it to him every other day.

(122)   *Social Worker*: And [he] possibly may have a hostile wife who, uh, maybe is dissatisfied with what he's, his behavior, and isn't willing to give it to him.

(123)   *Psychiatrist*: Yeah. I think we should think about those things, but I don't think we should put them down as facts.

The use of past records in present theorizing seemingly implies faith in the accuracy of the records. An independent coding of team members' opinions about the patient records revealed that this was indeed the case.[3] The members of most teams suggested that the records were "very helpful," "amazingly good," or "quite accurate." Some indicated surprise that the records were so complete. Only three teams made negative or critical comments about the records.

   One of the "skeptical teams" was one of the two previously categorized as not collectively reviewing records prior to interviewing patients. The other two were those categorized as "less theorizing." These teams reviewed records in a manner resembling more the simple "notation of data" than the elaborate "construction of theory." This is not to say that no inferences were made during the record-reading. Team members were occasionally observed making hypothetical inferences. For instance, during the reading of records, one psychiatrist would consistently nod his head "as if a picture of the patient was falling into place." A few times this same individual displayed his present-tense "summary judgments" to other members (for example, "Troubled and angry in here. And he looks like he's got it all resolved"). These public displays, however, were infrequent and less elaborate than the "theory-building" evidenced by the seven theorizing teams.

   Other signs of preinterview theorizing were also minimal. Both teams (F and C) made numerous references to patients' physical appearances in the official photograph accompanying the record. In interviews and postinterview discussions, however, members commented that the patients frequently looked better or at least very different from what they expected them to look like. These references indicate some selective expectations through previewing. Some of this would seem to be inevitable. The important difference between these teams and most others, however, was the infrequency of publicly displayed and collaboratively constructed interpretations of what the patient was really like.

   The "skeptical teams" displayed little in the way of preinterview theorizing. What they did display was a critical view of the records as "objective accounts" of a patient's past history. The following excerpt is typical of this generally negative attitude.

Excerpt 7-13. From Patient Review 102, Team F

(The psychiatrist is commenting on a report of a hospital staff psychologist.)

(5)   *Psychiatrist*: This whole damn report. This much is his observation of the patient. This much, uh . . . there's no results. You don't need to look at anything.

(6)   (All three members laugh.)

(7)   *Psychologist*: There's nothing there?

(8)   *Psychiatrist*: I'll tell you, there's one paragraph of results. The rest is his "what did the guy look like," which we know. We don't need that from the psychologists.

In interviews, the "skeptical" members expressed the belief that while they attended to data in the past record, they placed little trust in the "inferences and judgments" included therein. One respondent mentioned that a particular record had labeled a patient suicidal because it was said that he had "eaten glass" and "set himself on fire." In the course of its interview, however, the review team "discovered" that these "suicidal gestures" were actually stunts learned by the patient in his past job with the Barnum and Bailey Circus. According to the team, such stunts were performed by the patient in order to entertain others and attract attention. None of this was mentioned in the past record, which was said to contain but "a scarcity of data."

In summary, we have suggested that most teams display considerable preinterview theorizing in their treatment of patients' past records. This theorizing is filtered by such things as members' stocks of typical clinical interpretations and contrasts with previous patients. The three teams which showed little or none of this theorizing were also those which were most skeptical of the past records. Most teams were not. They found no difficulty in selectively previewing a patient's present through inferences from the past. This process of preinterview theorizing concludes the first major step in the social construction of patients' psychiatric realities.

## Notes

1. Two teams (K and H) did not collectively review the record before interviewing patients. One of these, however, had one member privately assess the record prior to the interview. Observations revealed that the "knowledgeable" member's questions were often phrased as hypothetical tests of inferences drawn

from the past record. This observation was corroborated by statements often made by the "knowledgeable" member in postinterview discussions. Frequently, this member would explain the "theoretical" basis of certain previously asked questions in light of information presented in the record. Furthermore, during interviews, the members of this team pointed out that the job of the "knowledgeable" member was to

just sort of listen to see if there was a correlation between what was being said and what was in the record. The person who read the record asked more specific kinds of questions during the interview, but only after the other two members would extract the history, etc., from the patient. Then [the knowledgeable] person could clarify how the patient was expressing the problems and see if there was a relationship to what the patient was saying with what was in the record.

2. By "past abstractions" we imply a concept akin to Schutz's idea of sedimentations of "second hand" knowledge. These form an important part of the complex stocks of knowledge required by modern consciousness. In so much as they are "within restorable reach," these sedimentations can be contextually displayed as "indexical resources" in supporting or challenging a particular "documentary interpretation." Cf. A. Schutz and T. Luckman, *The Structures of the Life-World* (Evanston, Ill.: Northwestern University Press, 1973).

3. The categorization of teams according to those evidencing considerable preinterview theorizing was done by the principle investigator. This categorization was based on an analysis of tapes and transcripts. The coding of members' opinions about the records was performed by a research assistant. This coding was based strictly on members' interview responses.

# 8

## Interviewing Patients: Conversational Features of Diagnostic Interviews

*The psychotherapist poses the questions; the patient answers. The psychotherapist then has the answers at his disposal. He may approve or disapprove, accept or reject, or merely ignore them. Throughout the entire interview, the psychotherapist is in complete control of the situation.*

> Thomas J. Scheff, "Negotiating Reality: Notes on Power in the Assessment of Responsibility," *Social Problems* 16 (Summer 1968): 13-14.

The sociological properties of talk between patients and diagnosticians during psychiatric interviewing differ significantly from those which characterize routine conversation between other actors in everyday life. In this chapter, we shall contrast the cognitive style of diagnostic conversations with that associated with everyday, ordinary, or mundane talk. The chapter will conclude with a substantive consideration of conversational practices employed by Lima review teams in interviewing patients.

### The Cognitive Style of Diagnostic Interviewing

Much ethnomethodological research has attempted to explore the importance of talk as a vehicle for producing an unproblematic sense of everyday social reality. In talk, actors typically produce and sustain the experience of what Schutz referred to as "the world of everyday life."[1] In conversing with one another, actors accomplish a sense of social life as a prestructured or preexistent objectivity which is both taken for granted and intersubjectively shared with others. Much of the early work of Garfinkel, Cicourel, Sacks, and others may be understood as attempts to describe the manner in which actors ongoingly produced a sense of this "life world."[2] Interactional or interpretive practices which establish a "sense of social structure" were noted and discussed. These included such practices as "the reciprocity of perspectives," through which one assumes that the other would see things in essentially the same way as oneself if self and other could change places; the "et cetera" practice, which entails glossing over or filling in ambiguous or vague utterances; and the use of "normal forms" by which actors cognitively restore congruity between contradictory accounts or perceptions.

Unlike everyday conversation, the talk occurring during psychiatric interviews is not geared toward producing a sense of the life world. Its purpose is not, in Schutz's sense of the term, "pragmatic." It is not directed at "getting by" or working with others to accomplish senses of prestructuredness, taken-for-grantedness, and intersubjectivity.[3] Its purpose is instead "applied theorizing." It is directed at explanatory and predictive discoveries about patients as objects of applied or clinical science. Patients are spoken to and heard, not as existential subjects with whom one must reckon, but as relatively disinterested objects about which one must make certain classificatory judgments.

Our distinction between the "pragmatic" motive of everyday talk and the "theoretical" motive of interviewing talk is, of course, ideally typical. Inasmuch as diagnostic interviewing is clearly consequential for the actors involved, we have chosen to describe it as applied, rather than purely theoretical. Nonetheless, during interviews, diagnostic agents appear to approach patients more as disinterested objects for theoretical dissection than as existential partners in pragmatic reality construction.

The verbal images produced by patients are not heard as necessarily participating in prestructured objectivity. They are not taken as corresponding to realities that exist before and independent of patients' descriptions of them. They may, in other words, be nothing more than patients' illusionary talk.

Patients' statements are not taken for granted as accounts of things as they really are. Instead, they are to be treated as possible projections of things as they "unreally" exist in the minds of the mentally ill. So too is intersubjectivity placed into question. In diagnostic interview talk, one does not assume a reciprocity of perspectives or the belief that the consciousness of the other is like ours until further notice. Notice has already been given. One doubts that the other sees things the way he does. The purpose of interviewing talk is to diagnose differences rather than assume sameness.

The pragmatic interpretive procedures associated with everyday talk (that is, reciprocity of perspectives, et cetera, normal forms) are infrequently displayed in interviewing talk between diagnosers and patients. This should not be surprising, given the relatively theoretical focus of this talk. Rather than conceiving of patients as reciprocating others, diagnosers approach patients as possible producers of nonreciprocal illusion, delusion, or pretense. Rather than glossing over or filling in patients' statements, diagnosers routinely point out discrepancies and ambiguities. Rather than normalizing incongruities, diagnosers "stress" patients so that potential contradictions will emerge for all to see. Instead of "working with" patients to produce the appearance of a world held in common, diagnosers "work on" patients to produce the appearance of a world inhabited but not shared.

The treatment of patients and their talk as objects for theoretical scrutiny is not always manifest in the overt conversational exchanges of a given psychiatric interview. Often questions are asked and answers "apparently" heard as valid descriptions of a world of reality assented to by both parties. However, a comparison of these question-answer sequences with members' subsequent postinterview interpretations reveals that patients' answers are not often taken for granted as valid accounts.

The following excerpt presents an illustration of this process of nonreciprocal interpretation. A patient is asked to describe "people who had it in for him." On the surface the psychologist appears to accept the patients' account of being railroaded by a particular psychiatrist. In actuality, what team members are hearing is evidence of the patients' paranoia. There is no assumption that patient and team would reciprocally see things the same if they could change places. The possibility that the patient may have been railroaded is not attended to. This patient's past record has indicated paranoia as a problem. The "fact" of his paranoid thinking is attended to. This is evidenced by the interpretation given to this conversational sequence once the patient has left the room. Clearly team members were not working to achieve a sensed reciprocity of perspectives.

Excerpt 8-1. From Transcript of Patient Review 362

(238)   *Psychologist*: I know you were feeling that maybe the psychiatrists and some other men helped to railroad you.

(239)   *Patient*: Well, he told me he was going to give me a good report.

(240)   *Psychologist*: How do you know he didn't?

(241)   *Patient*: In the court he said they were going by his report.

(242)   *Psychologist*: And what did he say about you? Do you know anything particular?

(243)   *Patient*: No, not particular.

(244)   *Psychologist*: But you think he must have had it in for you because they went ahead and they sentenced you?

(245)   *Patient*: Yes.

(246)   *Psychologist*: Anybody else who had it in for you [pause]? Or disappointed you in the same way?

(247)   *Patient*: I don't think so.

(After the interview ends and the patient leaves, his answers are reinterpreted by team members. This reinterpretation is summarized by the psychiatrist and becomes part of the patient's permanent record.)

(305)   *Psychiatrist*:. . . The defendant did express several times what appeared to us as somewhat of a paranoid flavoring in his answers, especially regarding the psychiatrists who treated him before or here, and how he was dealt with in court.

The sequence presented above gives the impression that members talk deceptively to patients, that they appear to take a patients' account at face value when, in fact, they interpret the account quite differently. Actually, this sequence simply serves to document the observation that patients are "worked on" (as objects of theoretical interest) rather than "worked with." Occasionally this "working on" is manifested during the interview. Sometimes patients are actually talked about as topics of analytic interest, even as they sit, present to members' theorizing. This talking about patients as if they were nonhearing objects for investigation is illustrated in the following excerpt.

Excerpt 8-2. From Patient Review 162, Team H

(385)    *Psychiatrist*: Do you ever read any magazines or journals?

(386)    *Patient*: Yeah. My dad works at a store. He brings home some.

(387)    *Psychiatrist*: Mmm. [Question directed toward social worker rather than patient.] I was too much occupied by his records. I didn't pay attention. I don't like to ask the same question. Did you ask him about hallucinations?

(388)    *Social Worker*: Mmm, hmm. Yeah.

(389)    *Psychiatrist*: About any suicide attempts?

(390)    *Social Worker*: I didn't ask him that.

(391)    *Psychiatrist*: [Now turning to patient]: This is a dirty question. Did you ever try to kill yourself?

Talking about a patient when he or she is present is a clear example that team members do not assume a reciprocity of perspectives between themselves and patients. Patients are put in the position of being objects rather than participants in talk. Sometimes, however, the object status of patients comes as a surprise to patients themselves. In the following excerpt, the patient is initially addressed as if he were a coparticipant in talk. He is asked to tell a joke. After the completion of the joke, the patient is rudely awakened to the fact that his descriptions were not being taken literally by team members. His joke was not heard as a joke at all. What he thought was joke-telling was heard as personality-revealing talk. As the psychiatrist informs the naive patient: "The joke that you told has something to do with the way you feel about yourself."

Excerpt 8-3. From Patient Review 423, Team B

(168)    *Psychiatrist*: Do you like to tell jokes? Can you think of any jokes?

(169)    *Patient*: I don't really know [pause]. I hear a lot of Polack jokes from Mr. [name], one of the attendants.

(170)    *Psychiatrist*: Can you think of one?

(171)    *Patient*: Yeah. I can. You want to hear it [laugh]? This is funny. This Polack bought this bird dog and took it out one day. And came back and took it

out again. And one Polack said to the other that if that dog don't fly tomorrow I'm going to shoot him right on the ground. So much for the Polack joke. Hope none of you are Polish.

(172)    *Psychologist*: Would it matter? How much would it matter?

(173)    *Patient*: Well, I don't want to hurt nobody's feelings.

(174)    *Psychologist*: Well, you didn't ask first, though. You asked later.

(175)    *Patient*: That's another thing I do. You know, sometimes I say something, and stop and think that wasn't a very good thing to say.

(176)    *Psychologist*: Feel embarrassed now? Your ears are turning a little red.

(177)    *Patient*: No, not embarrassed, a little idiotic that you wanted me to tell these jokes. But I guess you're just trying to make me feel comfortable.

(178)    *Psychiatrist:* No. I'm not trying to make you feel comfortable. People, uh, the kind of jokes that people think or tell or enjoy helps me to know something about them . . . [pause]. The joke that you told has something to do with the way you feel about yourself. The dumb Polack joke. You refer to yourself as a dumb hillbilly?

The preceding excerpt illustrates to the patient and to us alike that diagnostic interviewers suspend the everyday conversational practice of assuming a "reciprocity of perspectives." It also illustrates a suspension of the everyday practice of trying to normalize incongruities. Rather than normalizing the embarrassing situation, the review members appear to press embarrassment as an issue in its own right. This is a typical practice observed in numerous interviews. In this instance, members are very emphatic about denying the patient his own attempt to normalize the situation. The patient suggests that he is aware that members are only trying to make him better. The psychologist quickly blocks this normalizing effort. "No. I'm not trying to make you feel comfortable," he responds. "People, uh, the kind of jokes that people think or tell or enjoy helps me to know something about them."

Glossing and filling-in-meaning practices are also typically excluded from diagnoser-patient talk. When one patient said that he had erotic dreams about being with a woman, a diagnoser returned with a question asking the patient to be more specific. "Being with a woman? In what way? What exactly do you mean?" Patients' statements are not allowed to pass easily. They are liable to be returned to the patient for further elaboration. A patient who disclaimed being a homosexual was asked: "Tell me, what is a homosexual?" Diagnosers press their search for exactness by challenging single words or phrases that would likely be glossed over in most everyday talk. Note, for instance, the way a patient is called into question for using the term "mostly at night" (line 76) in the following excerpt. The term is not glossed over, but challenged.

Excerpt 8–4. From Patient Review 100, Team F

(The patient has been talking about the kinds of voices that he hears in his dreams. These voices were said to usually concern "pretty ideas." The patient admitted, however, that occasionally these dreams would frighten him. In the following sequence, the psychiatrist probes for evidence of daytime voices.)

(75) *Psychiatrist*: I'll bet they did. How about the voices during the daytime? What are they like?

(76) *Patient*: I don't hear any in the daytime, mostly at night.

(77) *Psychiatrist*: You said "mostly," so there are some during the day, huh?

Along with negating the use of reciprocity of perspectives and "et cetera" practices, diagnostic interviewers also curtail the use of various normalization techniques. "Slips" of the tongue or any other parts of the body become noticed as topics for public scrutiny. "I notice that your hand is kind of shaking while we're talking." "Your ears are red. Are you embarrassed?" Observations and inquiries such as these are used to put the patient on the spot. Statements are made so as to probe for how a given patient reacts to stressful input. Attempts are made to challenge rather than save a patient's face (in Goffman's sense of the term). Normalization is denied rather than practiced. As with a nonreciprocity of perspective and the disuse of "et cetera" practices, this feature of psychiatric interview talk contributes to the theoretic critique rather than to the pragmatic construction of a patient's sense of social reality.

In the preceding discussion, we have noted several differences between the cognitive style of interview talk and that of everyday life. These differences have been described in terms of such features as the nonreciprocity of perspectives, the disuse of "et cetera" practices, and a reluctance to normalize discrepant forms. Each of these differences appears to be grounded in the distinction between the applied theoretical commitment of interview talk and the pragmatic commitments of talk in everyday life. In the following section, we shall outline several substantive features of the applied theoretical talk that occurred between diagnosers and Lima State patients.

## Substance of Diagnostic Interview Talk

In considering the substance of talk during diagnostic interviews, we shall attend to five items. These include the conversational practices whereby members pursue selective question-answer sequences; the tendency for members to offer patients explanatory accounts of their own behaviors; the process of "selective hearing"; disciplinary differences arising in the use and allotment of interview talk; and the presentation of various diagnostic identities by patients in the process of talking with diagnosticians. In each of these areas we shall examine the properties of diagnostic interview talk as they contribute to the construction of definitions of patient's psychiatric realities.

## Pursuing Selective Questioning

Through their selection of questions, team members generally defined the substantive parameters of a given diagnostic interview. Questions were frequently geared toward confirming or validating an impression that members had of patients from having read their past records. In addition to this "theory-pushing" style of questioning, members also routinely engaged in what might be called "theme-pushing." By this, I mean that members searched for documentation on certain clinical themes regardless of the nature of a patient's case or charges. For instance, some clinicians were always pushing for patients to show "insight" into their past behaviors. Others appeared more concerned with displays of "responsibility" or attitudes toward sexual behavior. Examples of both "theory-pushing" and "theme-pushing" will be considered in the following excerpts.

Theory-pushing question-answer sequences are usually grounded in members' preinterview theorizing about a patient's problems. In a case where members had previously "discovered" that a patient's aggressive behavior was linked to a "bad home situation" a social worker opens an interrogatory sequence with the following statement.

Excerpt 8-5. From Patient Review 440, Team D

(The patient has just stated that, although he has ten brothers and sisters, "I got along pretty good. Got along with everybody." The social worker does not accept this as an answer and rephrases his inquiries so as to "expose" the real problems the individual must have had at home.)

(117) *Social Worker*: Do you want to tell us about your family background?

(118) *Patient*: There ain't much to tell.

(119) *Social Worker*: Well how did you get along with them?

(120) *Patient*: I got along pretty good. Got along with everybody.

(121) *Social Worker*: Big family you have. You have eleven brothers and sisters?

(122) *Patient*: No. Just ten.

(123) *Social Worker*: Ten of you, then? Eleven children altogether. You were what, which number, which child?

(124) *Patient*: Fourth one.

(125) *Social Worker*: Fourth one, fourth oldest?

(126) *Patient*: Yeah.

(127)   *Social Worker*: I imagine it was a pretty hard cost of living with so many people around. Left pretty much by yourself to take care of yourself and so on. Can you describe how you got along with your brothers and sisters and your parents?

In the preceding sequence the social worker's prior assumption that family problems are the patient's problem leads to the rejection of the original "I got along" answer and a rephrasing of the original question. In the ensuing conversation the social worker gets the patient to admit that he fought with his brothers and sisters and that his mother and father fought occasionally. These are the types of answers that the social worker recognizes as fitting what the team already knows about the patient. In each subsequent inquiry, the team expanded the range of negative family information being gathered. When the patient stated that his father worked all the time, a team member responded: "Yeah, that's what I thought. How often is he at home? Or [did he] work all day? At nights too?" After the patient stated that his parents, who "got along pretty good," only fought once in a while, a team member asked: "What'd your mother and father argue about when they argued?" Thus even potentially positive responses were probed until some negative features emerged. Members appeared committed to verifying their theoretical inferences about the patient's life. When the patient responded that he was out of the house during most times that his parents would "get into it," the team's psychiatrist followed with another attempt to document the problematic nature of the parental relationship. "But there was [sic] quite a bit of these fights," suggested this diagnostician. "They'd argue about a lot of things?"

A further example of "theory pushing" is presented in the following excerpt. In both cases it is evident that the team member's fellow diagnosticians are the real audience for the questioning. A patient's answers are heard as data to be related to prior theorizing. In the first excerpt the team has already categorized the patient as a manipulative psychopath. When the patient states that he knows better than to get caught fighting on the streets his words are interrogatorily dissected so as to reveal his manipulative nature. What he is "really" saying is that he'll attempt to disguise his future deviant behavior.

Excerpt 8-6. From Tanscript of Patient Review 432, Team B

(The patient has just stated that he now knows better than to get involved in trouble again.)

(116)   *Psychologist*: You'll know better? You know better now?

(117)   *Patient*: Know better than to get caught fighting on the streets.

(118)   *Psychologist*: And you'll go somewhere where you won't get caught?

(119)   *Patient*: No. I ain't going to be fighting no more.

In addition to theory-pushing it has been suggested that "theme-pushing" occurs routinely in the course of a diagnostic interview. In interview after interview certain team members push themes that appear to be related to their particular clinical orientation. For instance, one psychiatrist repeatedly demanded that patients demonstrate insight into the nature of their problems. In the subsequent team member interview, this same clinician described himself as an eclectic who places considerable emphasis on a patient's development of insight. Notice his interrogatory demand for insight in the following question-answer sequence.

Excerpt 8-7. From Transcript of Patient Review 362, Team L

(The patient has been talking about his past charges for threatening his ex-wife.)

(139)    *Psychiatrist*: Why do you feel so intent about threatening her?

(140)    *Patient*: I don't know. Always around Christmas time it happens. I miss the family and . . .

(141)    *Psychiatrist*: And you say you don't have emotional problems? I didn't say you were mentally ill. We all as human beings can have emotional problems. You certainly have displayed much of this. How do you feel?

(142)    *Patient*: I guess I do.

(143)    *Psychiatrist*: I'm not trying to convince you of it. I'm asking you to think. Because when a person begins to react that way, something is bothering them enough to do something to land you here.

A second example of "theme pushing" concerns a social worker who regularly attempts to elicit statements concerning responsibility for one's behavior. In our interview with this clinician, he revealed a commitment to a social or interactional perspective which places considerable emphasis on assuming responsibility. In the following excerpt the insistance on responsibility prevents the glossing over of the patient's statement about "finding someone to keep him in line."

Excerpt 8-8. From Transcript of Patient Review 441, Team D

(291)    *Patient*: I'd like to get married, find someone who'll keep me in line.

(292)    *Social Worker*: Keep you in line? Why can't you keep yourself in line?

(293)    *Patient*: I could keep myself in line but I think I'll probably need some help on. . . .

(294)    *Social Worker*: See, nobody can make you do anything. We make ourselves do things. People, there's ideas, maybe, but. . . how would you do that? How would you do that, keep yourself in line?

In the preceding excerpts the commitment of clinicians to certain perspectives (that is, searches for insight and responsibility) resulted in raising issues that other clinicians may have let pass. It is in this manner that general theoretical dispositions channel themselves into specific diagnostic interactions. The disposition of the clinician functions, as it were, alongside theories gleaned from the past record as another indexical determinant of the direction that diagnosis may take. It further provides selective structure for question-asking and answer-hearing. It contributes to an image of psychiatric decision-making as an inherently contextbound process, rooted more in the sense-making practices of clinicians than in the discernible behavior of patients.

**Offering of Explantory Motives**

In managing question-answer sequences, team members often appeared to offer patients explanatory accounts of their past or present behaviors. These accounts ordinarily coincided with members' emerging theories about why patients acted in this or that way. How patients responded to such offerings was an important determinant of how they would be viewed by team members. Patients who accepted and/or elaborated upon members' offerings were likely to be viewed as possessing insight. Those who resisted the interpretive direction suggested by members' questions were likely to be viewed as lacking insight or not understanding the motives underlying their behavior. This offering of explanatory accounts is illustrated in the following excerpts. In the first instance, the diagnostician offers a convicted rapist an explanatory account of his motives in terms of "being scared of girls." In the second, the team offers the patient an account of his exhibitionism in terms of "getting back at his father." In both cases, the patients reject or resist a team's theoretical offerings. In both instances the team eventually decides that these patients have little or no insight into their own behavior and continue to be psychopathic offenders who may repeat the crimes for which they are presently confined.

Excerpt 8-9. From Transcript of Patient Review 440, Team D

(In this sequence the social worker appears to be offering a patient an account of his behavior in terms of being afraid of girls. When the patient seemingly rejects this account, the team member continues his selective probe in order to display that, despite the patient's disavowal, this "rapist" has had problems relating to women.)

(305)   *Patient*: I was just driving around, you know, and I was going home. I think I was. And I saw this girl coming down the road, you know, so I tried to pick her up and put her in the car, you know. She started screaming and running and I couldn't catch her, so. . . .

(306)   *Social Worker*: How about guys?

(307)   *Patient*: I don't mind guys any.

(308)     *Social Worker*: Well, what makes a difference, do you think?

(309)     *Patient*: I don't know.

(310)     *Social Worker*: You keep telling yourself that maybe you're scared to talk to girls, something terrible might happen to you if you talk to them?

(311)     *Patient*: I ain't saying that.

(312)     *Social Worker*: How did you get along with your sisters?

(313)     *Patient*: I guess good.

(314)     *Social Worker*: Did you seem to fight more with them than you did with your brothers or less?

(315)     *Patient*: Less.

(316)     *Social Worker*: Did you talk with your brothers more than your sisters, or talk with your sisters more than your brothers?

(317)     *Patient*: Talk with my brothers a lot.

Excerpt 8-10. From Transcript of Patient Review 443, Team D

(The team has already articulated the "theory" that the patient's problems with exposing himself are tied to his anger and resentment toward his father. In this excerpt they offer this account to the patient as an explanation of his behavior.)

(238)     *Social Worker*: If you were to look back at all the things you've done, that you've been arrested for and so on, would you say any of them got you, uh, did something for you in terms of getting back at your father [pause]?

(239)     *Patient*: Mmm, let me see if I understand your question. You're saying that uh, uh, does any of these crimes that I've done have effect with my father?

(240)     *Social Worker*: Yeah, uh, where at one time you said. . . .

(241)     *Psychologist*: Did you feel like you were getting even?

(242)     *Social Worker*: . . . You know—like "I'll get back at you, you bastard, and then go out and do something to show him up or make him feel bad or. . . .

(243)     *Patient*: No. No. No. The only time with my father was just to show him that I could defeat him.

The preceding excerpts illustrate cases in which members' offerings of explanatory accounts are rejected by patients. In such instances, team members quickly change the topic to other areas of inquiry. In subsequent postinterview discussions, patients' answers are cited as reflecting such things as denial, rationalization, or the lack of insight. When patients accept members' offerings, the reverse occurs. Members stretch out the theory-confirming question-answer sequences and cite these as signs of a patient's strength. Note how patient's acceptance of a psychiatrist's theorizing is taken as a document of insight in the following interview sequence. The psychiatrist's lengthy offering is clearly on invitation for the patient to accept a particular theoretical explanation of his own psychiatric reality.

Excerpt 8-11. From Transcript of Patient Review 360, Team L

(The patient in this case is a convicted rapist whose crimes all occurred while intoxicated. The psychiatrist is offering a "deeper" explanation of the patient's problems. He is suggesting that there must be an "underlying reason" for the patient's behavior. He is making it clear that the influence of alcohol will not be heard as an "acceptable account".)

(109)   *Psychiatrist*: I wonder, Mr. 360, if you have thought about it. You might have thought about it and might not have given it too much meaning. Or you have not thought about it. But I think it is for your benefit. Very important. If I understand your expressions correctly, I have the feeling that you honestly believe that the reason why you are here is because of alcohol. That may have been the conveyer. That may have been the one thing that allowed you or that happened at the same time. But I wonder if you have thought about the millions of people that do drink and do drink too much, a lot, and do not commit these crimes. For what I'm trying to help you, think about, is that when you drink, when your judgment is removed by alcohol, then you will act out something that is already there. There is your key—and there you will find answers.

(110)   *Patient*: Yeah, that's right. I go to group therapy here and we've talked about that at some lengths. And I don't know whether it's a crutch. You look back and say—"Yeah. I was drunk. I did this. I did, but maybe the thought was already there. But if I'm sober I don't act them out." Right?

(111)   *Psychiatrist*: Right! You're under control. I just wanted to bring this up for your thoughts and consideration and that you might seek specific help in helping to get rid of that particular problem.

In the preceding excerpt the patient both hears and accepts the psychiatrist's offered account of his own motives. After affirming the clinician's offering, he asked, "Right?" The diagnoser lets him know that his answer was appropriate. "Right! You're under control." In the postinterview discussion it is stated that "he certainly doesn't know all the things to say, but he sounds remarkably insightful and controlled." Through the management of interview talk the diagnostician was able to produce external "evidence" of a patient's "internal" mental status. As such, the offering of motives represents an important vehicle in the social construction of another's psychiatric reality.

**Selective Hearing of Answers**

In addition to selectively asking questions and offering explanatory accounts, review team members often appear to selectively hear a patient's response in terms of categories compatible with the direction of their own theories.

Sometimes this selective hearing takes the form of "re-forming" an incompatible interpretation into a compatible one. Other times it results in an apparent "mishearing" of what the patient actually said.

In the following excerpt I shall depict a typical example of selective hearing through "re-forming" a response. Team members have suggested that the patient is basically controlled by external stimuli and that this problem underlies his abusive use of alcohol. This use of alcohol was in turn associated with his past convictions for indecent exposure. Notice that when the patient states (in line 361) that he's "solved this problem" team members really hear him saying that he's just afraid of the consequences of getting caught (line 366). The ensuing question-answer sequence is managed by members so as to selectively validate this second hearing as the correct hearing. This hearing is accomplished by the selective manner in which team members publicly focus (line 367) and refocus (line 377) what the patient is "really" saying.

Excerpt 8-12. From Transcript of Patient Review 443, Team D

(The patient has been talking about what he has learned from his period of incarceration and hospitalization.)

(361)    *Patient*: I've solved this problem drinking, and I don't have to worry about drinking anymore.

(362)    *Psychiatrist*: Why are you so certain? Why are you so certain about that?

(363)    *Patient*: Because, well, I can say why, because, uh, there's several patients here they've slipped in wine and I could have set back there and participated with them drinking but I didn't. I didn't break no rules to the hospital.

(364)    *Social Worker*: What would have happened if you did drink the wine?

(365)    *Patient*: Because if I did drink the wine I would have felt that, you know, it would have brought me back to the stage of me drinking again and make me continue on doing this. And then I thought to myself right away, I said, now this is what I said to myself, I said, "Now look at it," I said. "Mr. [Patient 443], look at it this way. I'm married. I have three children. I have a good business. I got a good thing to work for," I said, "why should I let all this go down the drain?" This is what I thought. Before. . . .

(366)    *Social Worker*: You wouldn't get out, in other words, if you drank the wine here?

(367)    *Patient*: Please?

(368)    *Social Worker*: You wouldn't get out of here if you drank the wine here? Ended up with problems again, right?

(370)    *Psychiatrist*: Would that hold you back, too?

(371)    *Patient*: Please?

(372)    *Psychiatrist*: Would that hold you back, too, that they're going to keep

you longer or put you in another ward or unit or cell or something or give you a bad report, or. . . ?

(373)  *Patient*: Mm, well, uh, I would say you're asking me, uh, do I feel that it would, uh, in what manner are you saying?

(374)  *Psychiatrist*: Is that a deterrent, would that stop you from thinking about uh. . . .

(375)  *Psychologist*: That you might be ineligible to another reward or you might have to stay here longer if you were drinking.

(376)  *Patient*: Yeah, 'cuz I would be breaking the rules. Yes.

(377)  *Social Worker*: Yeah. If it was on the outside you might have taken a drink, but inside here, if you did, you know there's going to be some consequences to it.

In the preceding chain of questions and answers it appears that team members guide the patient's responses so that (in lines 376-377) they finally accomplish a "firm" sense that what they heard all along was what the patient was "really" saying (although not in so many words). The difference here is between what the patient "actually" was saying as opposed to what he "really" was saying. Team members heard the latter from the beginning. Through the chain of focused inquiries, members were able to elicit (or coax) an actual "saying" (line 377) from the patient which corresponded to what they were really "hearing" all the time.

The selective hearing by team members of real statements that were not actually expressed in so many words may be attributed to their special clinical "expertise." From another perspective it seems to reflect clinicians' development of theoretical categories into which statements by the patient are selectively fit. Sometimes this theorizing about a patient as psychiatrically disturbed can lead to actual "mishearings" of things said. Note how the following answers provided by patients are "misheard" to provide an additional documentation of trouble, negative evidence, or trauma.

Excerpt 8-13. From Transcript of Patient Review 50, Team B

(In this sequence, the psychiatrist mishears the patient's side about borrowing coffee as a possible document that the patient has trouble when others try to to borrow coffee from him.)

(144)  *Psychiatrist*: How have you been getting along with the other patients here?

(145)  *Patient*: Good. I've getting along with them good. As long as there are patients here who I can borrow coffee from I'll get along good. I even got some coffee but I only got one pack, two packs. I owed one pack to someone and, uh, the other pack only lasted me a day. It didn't last a day even.

(146)  *Psychiatrist*: A pack of what, is it?

(147)    *Patient*: A pack of coffee. So I have to borrow from other patients till it's time when I get my own coffee again. If I don't loan it out to someone else, I'll do OK.

(148)    *Psychiatrist*: Drink a lot of coffee?

(149)    *Patient*: Yeah, yeah.

(150)    *Psychiatrist*: When they do try to borrow your coffee, what happens?

(151)    *Patient*: I don't know. I must misunderstand your question.

(152)    *Psychiatrist*: You said you get along all right with all the patients as long as they don't try to borrow your coffee.

(153)    *Patient*: Oh, no, I didn't say that. I said as long as I can borrow coffee.

Excerpt 8-14. From Transcript of Patient Review 50, Team B

(Here again the psychiatrist mishears part of the patient's response. He mishears "an aid at a mental hospital" (possibly positive information) for "Aidat, the mental hospital" (possibly negative information).

(289)    *Psychiatrist*: Now one other thing that puzzles me is—you were out of school for about four years. What did you do during that time?

(290)    *Patient*: I worked in the Job Corps. I worked in the post office. I was a Coca-Cola route salesman. I was a clerk in a produce department of a shopping center of a grocery store chain. I was, I was an aid at a mental hospital for six weeks, and then I was a bus driver. . . .

(291)    *Psychiatrist*: Did you say you were in Aidat, the mental hospital?

(292)    *Patient*: No.

(293)    *Psychologist*: An aid.

(294)    *Psychiatrist*: Oh, an aid. Oh!

Excerpt 8-15. From Transcript of Patient Review 013, Team K

(The psychologist has been using the theme that the patient has no meaningful relationships with women. In accordance with this theme, he selectively converts hearing of "sister as visitor" into "sister as girlfriend".)

(150)    *Psychologist*: Does any girl come visit you?

(151)    *Patient*: Used to.

(152)    *Psychologist*: Used to?

(153)    *Patient*: My sister. My sister. I just had a visit.

(154)    *Psychologist*: So your sister is your girl friend?

(155)    *Patient*: No, I didn't say that—I didn't say my sister was my girl friend.

Excerpt 8-16. From Transcript of Patient Review 013, Team K

(The psychologist has been probing the patient about friendships he has developed in his twelve and one-half years in the hospital. The patient has responded by indicating how difficult it is to trust anybody within the hospital. When the patient describes Lima as a "jungle," however, the clinician appears to hear this as if the patient were speaking literally. In the same fashion he jumps to a selective hearing about the patient's listening to talk on or in the television.)

(150)  *Psychologist*: Do you have any enemies?

(151)  *Patient*: Not that I know of. Maybe. Maybe [unclear].

(152)  *Psychologist*: Uhum. Do you think, do you think that there's anybody here who's trying to harm you?

(153)  *Patient*: Well, uh, trying. It all depends on what you call harm.

(154)  *Psychologist*: Trying to do anything against you.

(155)  *Patient*: Somebody can give you a cigarette and try to con you out of something. This is a jungle.

(156)  *Psychologist*: This is a jungle, uh!?

(157)  *Patient*: No. This is an expression. You watch TV. You see people getting killed on the screen every day and you listen to the news.

(158)  *Psychologist*: People on TV talk to you?

(159)  *Patient*: I listen to them. I listen to you.

(160)  *Psychologist*: Do you talk back to them?

(161)  *Patient*: I would consider. . . .

(162)  *Psychologist*: Do you?

(163)  *Patient*: Not necessarily. I wouldn't call it talking back. [The patient then continues his explanation, suggesting that the kinds of talking to the TV he means involve things like trying to give the answers to game-show questions prior to the contestants.]

Selective hearing represents another interactional practice employed by clinicians in constructing documentation of a patient's problematic condition. In the preceding excerpts we have noted how members hear or even mishear patients' statements in such a manner as to interpret them with a negative or pathological twist. Along with the selective asking of questions and offering of accounts of illness, selective hearing facilitiates the construction, ascription, and defense of imputed deviant (mentally ill, dangerous, or psychopathological) identities.

### Disciplinary Differences between Team Members

Differences in members' disciplinary statuses were reflected in the substantive nature of their questioning. This was somewhat more the case of psychiatrists than it was for either psychologists or social workers. Interviews would ordinarily begin with a sequence of general inquiries into a patient's past history, present functioning, and future plans. Questions into these matters would be asked regardless of the disciplinary status of the examiner. Subsequent or follow-up inquiries were more specialized and reflected greater differentiation along disciplinary lines.

Psychiatrists routinely asked questions geared toward obtaining information about a patient's cognitive, emotional, and intellectual functioning. Clinical psychologists appeared most concerned about getting parents' verbal account of how they cognitively or emotionally related to this or that past or present situation. Social workers asked many questions about how environment, family, and work relationships. These differences appeared related to the disciplinary status of the asker. Yet, it is important to note that only psychiatrists had exclusive claim to a particular or specialized line of inquiry. Psychologists and social workers placed greater emphasis on certain themes. Members of all three disciplines, however, were observed inquiring into these areas at one time or another. On the other hand, psychiatrists appeared to have the exclusive prerogative in asking special questions about a patient's general cognitive orientation and emotional and intellectual functioning.

The specialized psychiatric line of inquiry was typified by relatively standardized or "packaged" questions, asked independently of a patient's particular problems and legal history. Questions asking the patient what day it was and what was the name of the current president or capital of the state appeared to be directed at ascertaining a sense of the patient's orientation to time and space. Questions asking the patient to perform relatively elementary mathematical operations were aimed at assessing intellectual competencies. In addition to these questions, patients were frequently asked to interpret proverbs or say what they would do in this or that hypothetical situation. Psychiatrists described such inquiries as means of obtaining information on patient's reasoning processes, possible retardation, and reality testing. Each of these lines of investigation appeared to be the prerogative of the psychiatrist.

During diagnostic interviews, the clinical psychologist appeared most concerned about getting patients' verbal accounts of how they cognitively or emotionally related to this or that past or present situation. "How did you feel at that time? Were you tense and uneasy? What was going through your head at the time? Do you feel nervous now?" These were all lines of inquiry more particular to the disciplinary domain of the clinical psychologist.

While psychiatrists' questions tended to focus on general orientation to reality and psychologists' inquiries emphasized internal reactions to particular situations, social workers asked many questions about home environment, family, and marital relations. Their inquiries were often grounded in a social theorizing which seemed to portray the individual as the product of parental and/or peer socialization. In addition to this "family history" emphasis, social workers also led frequent inquiries into patients' legal status.

154

The division in question-asking among disciplines seems to have been an emergent characteristic of the patient reviews. There is no evidence that teams deliberately organized their interviewing practices to provide such a division of labor. This division, nonetheless, enabled members to display their professionalism along the lines with which they are probably most familiar. The near exclusivity of the psychiatric line of inquiry, however, seems to afford these members with a symbolic resource by which to underscore their importance and/or indispensability to the work at hand. This status differential will be discussed further in our subsequent discussion of the role of power differences in determining the direction of psychiatric decisions (Chapter 9). For now it is enough to observe that disciplinary differences appear to be an essential variable in accounting for substantive differences in questions asked of patients.

**Patients' Presentation of Various Diagnostic Identities**

Much of the preceding discussion has focused on practices employed by team members to manage diagnostic conversations with patients. All of this does not imply, however, that team members are in total control of the situation or that psychiatric interviews are one-way streets in the labeling of deviants. Our own interviews with patients are also conscious of manging certain identities for presentation to the diagnosers. This idea, of course, has been suggested in previous research. In the case of the Lima reviews, however, certain patients referred to their attempts to figure out what team members wanted in the following manner.

Excerpt 8-17. From Comments of Lima State Patient Interviewed by Researchers after Patient Reviews

We did discuss it among each other—what you could expect when you went in there. Of course, when one guy goes in the next guy is going to ask you, "Well, what did they ask you?" You know. It's only natural to do that. And we did talk about it, but I didn't think they asked each individual the same questions. Because, simply because of your record. It's different. Each guy's record was different, and they, quite naturally, the questions tended to vary.

Although patients' management of a diagnostic identity is an important topic, it is not of central concern in the present analysis. We are more interested in how team members differentially handled various interactional postures presented by patients. Ours, after all, is essentially a study of social controllers rather than of the socially controlled. In general, patients are perceived as presenting one of three diagnostic faces. They either display, admit, or deny identities as psychiatrically troubled individuals. In the following paragraphs, we shall outline the different reactions of team members to each of these styles of patient presentation.

*Displaying Psychiatric Disturbance*

This mode of patient presentation does not involve self-evaluative statements on the patient's part. His or her behavior is taken by team members as sufficient evidence of the presence of illness. The issue of whether the patient thinks of him or herself as having psychiatric troubles is never raised. This is not to say that the patient is *really* ill. It is simply to say that what the patient does or says is enough for team members to see or hear that the patient is really ill. Although in a handful of cases a patient was said to actually experience audio or visual hallucinations, more commonly the patient was viewed as not being oriented to or able to coherently answer questions asked by team members. It is as if the logic of her or his response is not synchronized with the logic of members' questions.

An example of the "displaying" mode of patient presentation is illustrated in the following excerpt. The patient has been talking about what team members believe are "bizarre" topics. He has just discussed how he was an "air cleaner." According to the patient, this means "something like when you go to bed at night and you dream, and if you go to bed and don't dream, well, your head will be stopped up with a cold." When asked whether the past record was correct in stating that he had once talked to a doctor about having had babies, the patient responded by stating: "That's why I mean I didn't having anything to talk about then. Because, uh, he was talking about breeding different kinds of horses, and I didn't think the baby had anything to do with it." Responses such as this were not heard as "sane" answers to reasonable questions. These responses prompted the psychiatrist to confront the patient in the manner depicted in the following sequence. Through this confrontation the psychiatrist maneuvers the patient into partially assenting to a psychiatric definition of himself as a disoriented person.

Excerpt 8-18. From Transcript of Patient Review 100, Team F

(124)  *Psychiatrist*:  Mr. [Patient 100], I'm having a little problem I want to talk with you about. As we were talking, I'm having some problem in following all the things you are saying—in a straight line. Do you know what I mean? I'm wondering if you have that problem sometimes in thinking. Like sometimes you're thinking about one thing, and then your mind might jump to something else, because that's what it feels like to me.

(125)  *Patient*:  Yeah, that's happening too. My mind's going one way to get out of here. And I've been here eighteen years and nobody talked to me about getting a parole, you know. Nobody talked to me about getting out. . . .

(126)  *Psychiatrist*:  Let me—did you understand? My question was that I don't think, I know you want to get out, but I don't think you were asking it; let me try it again. Maybe I didn't make it real clear. When you're talking, OK. . . .

(127)  *Patient*:  OK.

(128)   *Psychiatrist*: Sometimes it seems to me like you, it skips around what you're talking about. You were talking about the air cleaner and horse breeding, et cetera. Now I wonder if sometimes your mind skips around, just the way it sounds when you talk?

(129)   *Patient*: Yeah.

(130)   *Psychiatrist*: So it's hard to concentrate.

(131)   *Patient*: Yeah, that's the way it go, that's the way it do. Skips and bounces all the time.

In the preceding excerpt, the patient appears to assent to the psychiatrist's description of his disoriented thinking. He offers nothing that can be categorized as deliberate resistance to the psychiatrist's interpretation. Nor does he directly admit that he has psychiatric problems. Unlike patients who offer admissions that they have problems (and need help), patients who simply display problems are not heard as having anything to say about themselves. Thier statements, rather than being about themselves, are heard as indicators of their (psychotic) selves. After members typify patients as presenting a "displaying mode" they quickly move to provide additional documents of his or her "bizarreness" and then proceed to terminate the interview. Nothing is believed to be gained from hearing more of what a patient has to say. All that has been learned has been in hearing how (disorientedly) things were said.

Once patients are fitted into the "displaying mode" team members routinely rely on psychiatrists to run through a series of general orientation questions in order to confirm their impressions of the patients. Exchanges such as the following are typical.

Excerpt 8-19. From Transcript of Patient Review 100, Team F

(The patient here is the same patient who "displayed" his disorientation in the previous excerpt.)

(210)   *Psychiatrist*: Let me ask you one question. Uh, let me ask you one little saying and you tell me what it means to you, OK?

(211)   *Patient*: All right.

(212)   *Psychiatrist*: It goes, "A rolling stone gathers no moss."

(213)   *Patient*: Wait, explain it again now.

(214)   *Psychiatrist*: "A rolling stone gathers no moss."

(215)   *Patient*: Well, I wouldn't say it doesn't. I'd say it gathers moss because, uh, we wouldn't have hailstones. I would say it was something like hailstones.

(216)   *Psychiatrist*: OK. Let me ask you, do you have any questions you want to ask us? We've asked you a lot? [The psychiatrist here begins to terminate the interview. The previous displays of the patient's "inappropriateness" have been confirmed by his "bizzare" interpretation of the proverb. The patient

has been confirmed in the "displaying mode." No more talk between clinicians and patient is needed.]

Patients in the displaying mode are characterized by team members in relatively neutral or objectlike language. Their illness has been discovered and documented. It is talked about as a thing which has a life of its own and which incapacitates the patient. The patient, however, is not spoken of in moralistic terms. He or she is portrayed as neither a "good" nor a "bad" actor. There is, in other words, little evaluation of the persons as a person, but considerable description of the person as an object of mental illness. This neutral talking about "displaying" patients is exemplified by members' making descriptive statements about the patient in terms of standard psychiatric nomenclature. It may be said, for instance, that the patient perseverates, shows concreteness, poor affect, looseness, or whatever. This "neutral" talk contrasts sharply with "moralistic" postinterview talk about patients who present themselves in either the "admitting" or "denying" mode. We shall elaborate upon this observation in our subsequent discussion of these other modes of patient presentation.

*Admitting Psychiatric Problems*

When a patient admits psychiatric problems, he or she makes self-evaluative statements without displaying particularly "inappropriate" behavior during the diagnostic interview. This mode of patient presentation is believed by team members to indicate a patient's insight into his or her own problems. The patient who can admit psychiatric problems is one who is generally believed to have problems but is also well on the way in controlling these problems. The following excerpts depict the accounting practices of patients who show "insight" by admitting their own problems.

Excerpt 8-20. From Patient Review 423, Team B

(The patient is a middle-aged male who was convicted of molesting a young girl and exposing himself to her. In the following sequence the patient admits the bizarreness of his actions and shows some insight into the causes for his disturbance-insight which coincides with the team's own pre-interview theorizing.)

(63)　*Psychiatrist*:　How about the charge?

(64)　*Patient*:　Well, I just received a, had a vasectomy, and, uh, it left me impotent. Is that what you call it?

(65)　*Psychiatrist*:　That's the word.

(66)　*Patient*:　And, uh, well, that's a pretty big shock, but it turned out it was only a temporary thing, which my doctor hadn't explained to me. Evidently

... it had me all shook up and I didn't know how to take it. I felt that I had to do something to prove myself that . . . this bizarre action, I guess.

Excerpt 8-21. From Patient Review 441, Team D

(Here the patient admits his past escapism and the abusive use of drugs. When team members press him to see if he is just making these "moral statements" to impress them—line 30—he responds "appropriately" by discussing the way he has personally been hurt by his past actions.)

(122)  *Psychologist*: So you start at what—about age fifteen?

(123)  *Patient*: Yeah, I had just turned fifteen.

(124)  *Social Worker*: You weren't getting much out of school. You didn't enjoy school, or it was boring to you, or what?

(125)  *Patient*: Well . . . at the age of fifteen, I didn't really enjoy it 'cuz I was more . . . I guess, rebellious against everything. I'd had a bad family life and just got in with the wrong friends and they were doing drugs and they had similar problems at home and we just got along, I guess [pause].

(126)  *Social Worker*: So, mainly it was to give you some laughs and make you feel good, at least.

(127)  *Patient*: To get away from the real facts of life.

(128)  *Social Worker*: What about now? How do you see it?

(129)  *Patient*: I see it as one big mistake.

(130)  *Social Worker*: You know we're not here to get you to make a moral statement. What's in it for you, really?

(131)  *Patient*: No. I know that. It was just a big mistake and I realize that now it was a bad mistake.

(132)  *Social Worker*: Why?

(133)  *Patient*: 'Cuz I'm here.

(134)  *Psychologist*: 'Cuz you got into trouble with the law?

(135)  *Patient*: Mmm, and, plus, I hurt myself doing it, taking drugs.

In discussing the "admitting mode" or self-presentation by patients, one additional qualification must be made. This concerns patients who insist that their problems existed only in the past and that they now have these problems under control. It seems that to be viewed as really admitting one's problems, one must see the connection between past and present problems. One must at least recognize that there are still some things to be worked on, problems that one is still not fully in control of. If patients persist in asserting that all their problems were in the past they are heard as "conning" or manipulating team members and are likely to be considered "psychopaths." In the normal flow of an interview, however, patients who initially admit only past problems are given the opportunity to show the "proper awareness" of problems that continue to exist. In the "vasectomy" case presented above, the patient is eventually maneuvered into recognizing that he still has personality problems associated with an inferiority complex. In the "drug user-escapist from reality case," excerpted thereafter, the individual is pushed to admit that he still needs help. This push to admit that the problem is still there is exemplified in the following excerpt, in which a team member is considerably more direct in getting an "admitting" patient to agree that his problem still exists.

Excerpt 8-22. From Transcript of Patient Review 366, Team L

(The patient has previously admitted emotional problems that were associated with his multiple acts of indecent exposure. In response to these admissions, the team psychiatrist stated: "You are very honest and we appreciate that. It has nothing to do with good or bad or right or wrong. But this is just to find out if you are aware, as we knew that this [the problem] was the case." In this excerpted sequence, the team is probing to see if the patient still recognizes that he has a problem.)

(119) *Psychiatrist*: You say now that you'll never do it again, but I know you will because you still have the problem. And that is why I'm going to tell you this. When and if you leave, it is your business to go and get psychiatric help and it's a very simple thing to correct. And as sure as you sit there you're going to do it again. You can get this corrected and get it over with.

(120) *Patient*: Sure.

(121) *Psychiatrist*: Because the next time you do it you aren't going to get out.

(122) *Patient*: Yes, sir.

(123) *Psychologist*: Doctor [psychiatrist's name], this is kind of a problem.

(124) *Patient*: My father said when I get out he can set it up with a psychiatrist.

(125) *Psychiatrist*: That's good. Because, you see, it's not because, you see, it's not because you want to or because we want to frighten you but because the problem is there and you happen not to know just why and you did those hundreds of times. You see what I mean.

(126) *Patient*: Yes.

(127) *Psychiatrist*: I know it's not very pleasant and we're not here for good or bad, right or wrong. OK? And you've been very honest when I asked you that question—and as sure as if you sit here you'll do it over and over again. So when you get out of here be sure to seek psychiatric help. Do you understand that?

(128) *Patient*: Yes. My father is going to set it up and pay for it until I get a job.

(129)  *Psychiatrist*: That's the only important thing there is—the greatest priority in your life.

(130)  *Patient*: Yes, sir, I know.

In discussing team members' views of patients in the "displaying mode," I have suggested that patients are considered in terms that are "morally" neutral. By this I simply mean that actors' behaviors are believed to be (more or less) totally controlled by the illness to which they are subject. They cannot, in other words, calculate the consequences of their actions. Such is not believed to be the case for patients in the "admitting mode." They are believed to have the insight to see the consequences of their behavior and recognize for themselves the problems that team members already recognize about them. Their actions, in other words, are seen to have a moral dimension. Moreover, they are perceived as sharing team members' definitions of their psychiatric troubles. They are viewed as "good" actors and talked about in terms that are "morally positive." Members typically speak of them as having various strengths, as manifesting a positive desire to improve themselves and as being well motivated. These sentiments are routinely expressed in postinterview discussions. As members commented (in one of the cases excerpted above): "Yeah, as I was saying, this guy seemed to be motivated. I don't think he's trying to play anything over on anybody. I just had to emphasize to him it would really be a good deal for him to continue some kind of out-patient therapy."

Positive postinterview comments about patients' personal strengths are one indicator that "admitting" patients are viewed in favorable moral terms by the review teams. A second indicator occurs within the structure of the diagnostic interview itself. The only cases in which clinicians talked with patients as reciprocating others (rather than merely using talk as a strategy to elicit psychiatric data) involved instances where a patient had first admitted having a problem. Such an admission, of course, served as an indicator that team and patient defined at least part of the social life in a similar fashion. In such instances, patients and team members occasionally "slipped" into normal conversation about such mundane matters as place of birth ("Oh, I knew someone who came from there."); speech patterns ("You know, you sound like my uncle. He was from the South, too."); hobbies ("Gee, my wife collects rocks, too. What kind do you collect?"); etc. Such "slips" would permit members and patients to (at least temporarily) establish a sense of an inter-subjective life world and provide them with a sense that certain things could (for the time being) be taken for granted. As an indicator of the significance of the "admitting mode" it is important to note that such slips were not observed in either of the other two major modes of patient self-presentation.

*Denying Psychiatric Problems*

Patients who deny having psychiatric problems are treated differently from those who display or admit problems. When patients deny a problem that team members seem sure that they have, members tend to push for admissions or agreement with clinicians' definitions of the situation. Patients were observed as presenting one of four strategies in response to this pushing. These strategies facilitated various degrees of negative attributions by team members. Each of these four responses will be examined in turn.

**Direct Resistance.** The first subtype of the denying mode involves patients who directly resist team members' definitions of the situation. Some patients are quite aggressive in their opposition to members' offerings. One such instance is presented in the following excerpt. The team has been trying to get the patient to see that he has a problem with freedom, that he is overrebellious. The patient attempts to turn the table on the team members in asserting that they, rather than he, are misperceiving what freedom is all about. This aggressive denial of members' definitions of the patient as having psychiatric problems earns him the negative evaluation of team members. After he leaves the room, members comment on his cockiness, stubbornness, and escapism. The diagnosticians do not believe what he was saying. They comment, instead, on how he was just "trying to impress" everybody. The following excerpt presents both his direct resistance during the interview and team members' subsequent interpretation of this behavior.

Excerpt 8-23. From Patient Review 361, Team B

(205) *Social Worker*: You ran away from the [school for delinquents] a lot of times. How come?

(206) *Patient*: Uh, the, uh, it wasn't like a school. It was like a jail. I mean you had to be here at a certain time, and there at a certain time, and, uh, I figure if you're born you should be free, right? And, uh, I don't know. I can't dig being congested in a confined area.

(207) *Psychiatrist*: You were allowed to be free until you did something that is not allowed.

(208) *Patient*: Uh, the thing is, uh, certain places like you, uh, you're allowed to be free as long as you sit and don't go over a certain boundary. But, uh, freedom doesn't have any boundaries.

(209) *Social Worker*: Did you do anything you wanted to?

(210) *Patient*: Not anything. I mean like, uh, there's laws.

(211) *Social Worker*: Aren't those boundaries?

(212)   *Patient*: But, uh, freedom extends beyond the boundaries like a bridge beyond them. You don't have to. . . .

(213)   *Social Worker*: You don't have to obey the laws?

(214)   *Patient*: You have to obey the laws, but you, uh. . . .

(215)   *Social Worker*: I thought you said they didn't matter.

(216)   *Patient*: I mean you go over them. . . .

(217)   *Social Worker*: You go over them, around them, around them, but at any rate you just avoid them.

(This exchange continues with the patient's refusing to yield his point and arguing that it is acceptable to break a law if "you don't concur with it" and that certain "laws are made to be broken." The interview concludes with the social worker's contending that he had never personally broken a law and the patient's replying, "That's kind of hard to believe 'cuz everybody's broken a law." The psychiatrist then thanks the patient and closes the interview. After patient 361 leaves the room, the team jumps on his aggressive denials and interprets his case in the following manner.)

(239)   *Social Worker*: The thing that he was saying that there's no need to break a law!

(240)   *Psychiatrist*: The more he went the deeper he got [laugh].

(241)   *Psychologist*: Oh, yeah, yeah. And he's just stubborn enough that he will not fall back.

(242)   *Psychiatrist*: I, I don't think I believe what he was saying. I was trying to impress how cocky I am or how I'm going to do anything and nobody's going to stop me. . . .

(243)   *Psychologist*: Right, right; on the other hand, I do think that his general orientation toward people is to feel that there is no functioning with them and have to get away from them, and it's tragic all the way around.

(244)   *Social Worker*: He can't have anything to do with people. Well, you got to consider with his social background. . . .

(245)   *Psychologist*: He needs treatment. He needs intense treatment.

(246)   *Psychiatrist*: I know, but that's a problem. I don't care what causes. . . .

(247)   *Psychologist*: That's right. And I think he should be kept here. . . .

**Denying through Detopicalization**: This form of resistance to members' formulation is less direct than the previous subtype of denial. In presenting this particular interactional face, patients sidetrack or derail the direction of team members' imputational inquiries. This detopicalizing is ordinarily achieved through the introduction of tangentially relevant, but essentially different, substantive materials. In the following excerpt, for instance, detopicalizing is achieved through first objecting to information being sought about one's parents. The patient reminds team members that he gave permission (for the researcher) to tape materials about him, but not necessarily about his parents. Later on the patient answers a question about hearing voices with the literal response, "I hear yours." This, of course, is not what team members were after. Nor is it exactly bizarre or disoriented talk. The detopicalizing patient is "technically" responsive to members' inquiries but is "in spirit" resistive to their efforts to ascribe a particular problematic identity.

Excerpt 8-24. From Transcript of Patient Review 013, Team K

(250)   *Psychologist*: Did your father get into trouble?

(251)   *Patient*: Not that I knew of.

(252)   *Psychologist*: Did he work?

(253)   *Patient*: Yeah, he worked. He raised eight kids. But he's retired.

(254)   *Psychologist*: What kind of work?

(255)   *Patient*: On the railroad.

(256)   *Psychologist*: Did your mother work?

(257)   *Patient*: I signed the paper. All this is going on tape. That ain't about me. You want to know about my daddy and mamma.

(258)   *Psychiatrist*: OK, Joe, OK. We understand that sometimes you hear voices.

(259)   *Patient*: Oh, uh, I hear yours. I'd hear it again if you asked me something else.

(260)   *Psychiatrist*: Well, sometimes though there might not even be people around and you hear voices.

(261)   *Patient*: Oh, uh, music. Like see that light [pointing to a light bulb in the distance]. If you were closer, it'd seem brighter. But you can't see it now. It goes with the voices. It's got to go somewhere. The wind's gonna take it somewhere. If you're in a locked cell, it's got to go somewhere. Somebody else—you can talk low, whisper but still someone's going to hear. When you speak of hearing voices, you can't hear but one at a time. If you hear all of them at the same time it would be a group. So how are you going to hear a voice? It would be a group talk.

(262)   *Psychologist*: So you hear a lot of voices?

(263)   *Patient*: No. No.

(264)   *Psychologist*: Joe, I was wondering, how did you get along with your dad?

Patients who detopicalize members' inquiries are viewed as indirectly denying their own illness. They are evaluated negatively by team members who comment on such things as their avoidance mechanism. The next subtype of denials represents, perhaps, a special variety of detopicalizing. Its users derail members' emergent imputations by presenting themselves as victims of the misdeeds or pathologies of others.

**Denying through Presenting Self as Victim**: Team members do not react sympathetically to patients who tell about the problems caused by others when they have been asked to describe their own problems. Patients who present themselves as victims rather than as problem persons are typically viewed as rationalizing and covering up their own disturbances. One male patient, for instance, related a story about being victimized by a "crackpot psychiatrist," by staff discrimination, and by the lack of treatment at Lima State Hospital. He characterized the home for delinquents which he attended as "more of a jail than a school." A sociologist who made such statements would hardly be viewed as psychiatrically disturbed (though she or he may be characterized as a bit radical). Moreover, similar statements had been given a clear factual basis in the investigations of Lima State Hospital that preceded the patient reviews. Nonetheless, the patient who uttered these remarks was viewed in quite negative terms. The diagnostic report for this nineteen-year-old male stated that "he rationalized considerably and left no doubt that he feels that he can handle the situation his own way, and that he's not agreeable to therapy and that he needs no help from anyone."

The "self as victim" mode of patient presentation does little to gain the sympathy of psychiatric diagnosticians. Another case illustrating the point involved the narrative of a patient who claimed to have been sexually abused at the hospital. Although this patient had, in fact, testified at public hearings on this matter, this narrative was heard as evidence of delusions and projections of the patient's own homosexual identity to others. In formulating its final opinion, the review team in question suggested that "some of this goes on but mostly it's just delusions." Again, the self as victim presentation is heard as evidence of further psychiatric troubles.

**Denying Although Nominally Assenting**: This final subtype of deniers included those patients who previously denied having particular psychiatric problems but, when pushed by team members, gave the appearance of agreeing with the clinicians' definitions of their problems. Unlike patients who "really" admit their problems, these "pseudoassenters" show no evidence of elaborating and incorporating members' ascribed psychiatric identities into their own stories. Those who were viewed as denying, although nominally assenting, were typically categorized as psychopaths or manipulators. The pushed "assentings" of two such deniers are presented in the following excerpts.

Excerpt 8-25. From Transcript of Patient Review 433, Team B

(The psychologist has begun this questioning sequence by suggesting that "they noted, they wrote in here every so often in your chart that you've been kind of a loudmouth, kind of a mean son of a bitch, as far as not caring, give people a lot of lip." In the subsequent series of inquiries and answers the patient indicates that actually he doesn't give anybody any trouble. He states that if others respect him, he respects them. He does indicate, however, that something that other patients occasionally say shows no respect for him. In the following sequence, the psychologist pushes for the patient to admit that he acts like a loudmouth when this particular thing is said.)

(195)   *Psychologist*: So what would you do if someone says that to you?

(196)   *Patient*: I just don't speak to them and I go on.

(197)   *Psychologist*: You don't mouth off?!

(198)   *Patient*: Yeah, I mouth off.

(199)   *Psychologist*: That's what I'm trying to get at. What might you say? None of your god-damned business or?

(200)   *Patient*: Probably.

(201)   *Psychologist*: Or what the fuck matter is it to you, or something like that?

(202)   *Patient*: Probably.

Excerpt 8-26. From Transcript of Patient Review 442, Team D

(The psychiatrist has been trying to get the patient to verbalize a statement about his problems. He has reminded the patient of his history of multiple arrests and has suggested that there must be some larger problem behind it all. In the following sequence the social worker seems to maneuver the patient into agreeing that susceptibility to peer influence—that is, "sort of a prestige thing"— must have been an underlying factor behind his crimes. The psychiatrist, however, challenges whether that is what the patient is "really" saying, asking: "Is that the way you felt or did he put some thoughts in your mind?")

(203)   *Social Worker*: Well, so if you got picked up as many times as the other guys that made you as good as the others?

(204)   *Patient*: Not really.

(205)   *Social Worker*: Well, I mean sort of a prestige thing, that uh, that everybody's doing it, getting arrested, and somebody who doesn't might be looked down on?

(206)   *Patient*: Well, it might be, in a sense. A person that might be tougher than everybody.

(207)   *Social Worker*: Everybody was boasting about getting arrested and thrown in jail and so on, or if it was a stolen car?

(208)    *Patient*: Mmmm. Yes.

(209)    *Psychiatrist*: Is that the way you felt or did he put some thoughts into your mind?

(210)    *Patient*: Well, uh, you know, as far as that goes, I was really then just like any other person. I would do things that anybody else would do.

In the preceding cases, as in those indicative of "the denying mode" in general, patients are responded to in "moralistic" terms as persons trying to "put something over" on the psychiatric team members. Thus, like patients in the "admitting mode," denying patients are believed to have some awareness of the consequences of their actions. Unlike admitting patients, however, they are construed as using this awareness for negative ends (that is, attempts at manipulating and disguising their "real selves" from team members). Paradoxically, this "negative" demonstration of awareness leads team members to suggest that these patients have no insight. They are usually believed to show signs of psychopathy along with any other illness they refuse to own up to. What all of this means, of course, is that to have insight (and to be morally evaluated in positive terms) is to draw agreement with members' definitions of one's problems. To act relatively rationally or calculably (that is, without the bizarre aspect of the "displaying" mode), but to deny members' ascriptions of one's problems, is to be seen as a "bad" actor.

The negative evaluation of deniers is situationally or indexically engendered. Clearly it depends more on the context in which something is said, rather than on its substantive content. Since members already "know" that the patient is disturbed, efforts to directly deny, detopicalize, or present one's self as a victim are all heard as efforts to skirt the "real" question. They are categorized as self-serving. Attempts at nominally assenting to members' definitions are viewed similarly. The timing of assent appears to be the important variable. In the last excerpt, for instance, certain substantive statements were made, which, in some other context, may have indicated a patient's insight into his or her problems (for example, line 201). Yet inasmuch as the patient had previously tried to deny his problems, these "revelations" are heard as further attempts to manipulate or impress team members. In the discussion following the interview with this patient, one member immediately comments that "I'm beginning to get worried with all of these guys wandering loose." It is then suggested that the patient was simply "trying to put his best foot forward" and that "manipulation is the name of the game." The moral ascription of a negative identity is evident in these summary phrasings by team members. Clearly, patients who present a denying mode are viewed in harsher terms than patients who "come off" in either of the other major modes of self-presentation.

*Summary*

In this chapter we have focused on the actual conversational exchanges occurring between team members and patients. We have described a cognitive style governing this diagnostic interview talk which distinguishes it from routine talk in the everyday world. Members' practices of pursuing selective answers, offering explanatory accounts, and hearing selectively were seen to contribute to the sense of the interview as a managed imputation of deviant identities. Disciplinary differences among team members were seen to make a difference in the substantive content of questions asked. Finally, differences among various modes of patients' presentation of themselves were discovered to be related to the manner and way that team members viewed patients as moral persons. In the next chapter we shall explore the manner in which all that emerges in preinterviews and interview theorizing is channeled into a single diagnostic construction of a patient's psychiatric reality.

**Notes**

1. Alfred Schutz, *Collected Papers I. The Problem of Social Reality* (The Hague: Martinus Nijhoff, 1962).

2. For an outline of these basic interpretive practices, see Aaron V. Cicourel, *Cognitive Sociology: Language and Meaning in Social Interaction* (New York: The Free Press, 1974). For an extended discussion of the "et cetera" practice and "glossing," see Harold Garfinkel and Harvey Sacks, "The Formal Properties of Practical Actions" in John C. McKinney and Edward A. Tiryakian, eds., *Theoretical Sociology* (New York: Appleton-Century-Crofts, 1970).

3. Probably the clearest statement of Schutz's position on these matters is found in his essay "On Multiple Realities," *Philosophy and Phenomenological Research* 5, 4 (1945): 77-97, reprinted in *Collected Papers I*, pp. 207-259.

**Deciding upon Psychiatric
Realities: Postinterview
Negotiations and the
Issuance of Final
Diagnostic Reports**

*The labels which we as observers confront are, so to speak, the end points of
much socially organized activity that enter into their production. To accept
such end points as points of departure for exploring the antecedent conditions
or independent variables that influence the labeling process is to neglect the
socially organized character of the labeling process itself. The question, then,
is how to transform the labeling process into an observable phenomenon to extract the rules that organize its assembly.*

> Alan Blum, "The Sociology of Mental Illness, in *Deviance and
> Respectability* (New York: Basic Books, 1970), p. 39.

At the end of the diagnostic interview, review team members typically thanked
patients for coming and explained that they would now discuss the whole case
and come up with a recommendation to the court. After the patient left the
room, teams entered into their final stage of their psychiatric decision-making—
the process through which final diagnostic statements are agreed to and made
public. Our consideration of this topic is three-fold. We shall first attend to the
"logical" procedures by which team members finalize their theories about
patients' psychiatric realities. We shall next consider several additional characteristics of psychiatric decision-making, which impact upon the substantive formulation of particular decisions. These characteristics include the manner in
which members negotiate displays of status and power, anticipate the consequences of making certain recommendations, and make practical use of
individual theorizing about deviance. The chapter concludes with an analysis
of methods employed to transform "ad hoc" clinical reasoning into "objective"
or "expert" findings.

**Finalizing Theories: Using Justificatory and Reconciliatory Logic**

Negotiations of final decisions were guided by two types of logic: a logic of
justification and a logic of reconciliation. The first arises insofar as most
clinicians had already developed a "sense of a decision" about a patient prior
to stating the decision in so many words. Often this decision (a particular
theoretical assessment of the patient's problem) is arrived at early in the review

169

process and subsequently elaborated and justified during the course of interviews and postinterview discussions. In the postinterview discussion, decisions (with which members have already been working) are publicly announced. Members then proceed to selectively summarize events and observations from the record and the interview that elaborate their reasoning and provide justification for what it is that they have already decided upon. This postdecision assembling of evidence we shall refer to as members' logic of justification.

The second form of logic employed by members arises from their need to view themselves as expert finders of facts, which exist independently of their own discovery practices. The team approach to diagnosis complicates the attainment of this end. In principle, each clinician could arrive at a theoretical understanding of the patient which contradicts the understandings of the other two. If this should happen, the "expertness" of one's fact-finding is placed into question and the "objectivity" of one's work is seriously challenged. The use of a set of logical practices which reconcile possible discrepancies and create the appearance of no serious disagreements among members allows members to avoid this discrepancy. These practices we shall refer to as members' logic of reconciliation.

## The Logic of Justification

In considering the review of psychiatric records, and the use of record data during diagnostic interviews, we observed that members make clinical "discoveries" about a patient's present through inferences derived from his or her officially defined past. This kind of "prospective" viewing of the patient appeared to be an intrinsic element of members' logic of discovery. In postinterview discussions this strategy is complemented by a kind of "retrospective" viewing. Once members announced their decision about a patient, numerous "facts" are retrospectively found to provide the grounds for recognizing that the announced decision is the right one. This "retrospection" is an intrinsic element of members' logic of justification.

The following excerpts exemplify members' retrospective logic of justification. The patient under consideration was typed as a sociopath during the review of his records and was said to be a "stone-cold" manipulator who "probably never got along with anybody." During the diagnostic interview members "managed" to sustain the direction of this theorizing. As soon as the patient left the room each member revealed that his or her decision was "in" on this individual. Members' evaluative comments were indicative that they still viewed the patient as a sociopath. In their subsequent exchanges, members cite a variety of evidence which supports their conclusion. His bottled-up hostility, welling-up eyes, his good looks, his age, his intelligence, and his desire to complete school are all taken as documents of his deviant identity. Members do not list all the evidence for and against a particular diagnosis. They already have their diagnosis; they already "know" the patient is a sociopath. What they do, instead, is retropsectively dig up information which supports their own theorizing and excludes other alternatives.

Excerpt 9-1. From Patient Review 422, Team B

(The assessment team begins the postinterview discussion by discrediting the patient's statement that he was too high to know what was happening when he slugged a guy in a grocery store. According to the team's psychiatrist, he was just "denying responsibility." It was further suggested that, although the patient interpreted his past behaviors as a way of getting back at his father, he really was not in touch with the true source of his hostilities.)

(149)    *Psychiatrist*: I guess he just couldn't.

(150)    *Social Worker*: I would too. His eyes were welling up there when you mentioned.... [The flow of the conversation is here interrupted for several exchanges by a question by the psychiatrist about why the record indicates that the patient is taller than he really is. The psychiatrist links this "mistake" to a probable fake report by the patient and continues the retrospective justification process by concluding: "He's always been a master liar."]

(155)    *Psychiatrist*: He's always been a master liar.

(156)    *Psychologist*: Uh-huh. Today I think you ought to take that into consideration. [The psychologist here appears to generalize to others so-called "psychopathic patients" whom the team will be seeing that day.]

(157)    *Social Worker*: [laughing]: A master liar!

(158)    *Psychiatrist*: Yeah. He's considered a real, uh.... He's a real con, uh ... he's a real con. He's used his good looks and that's what he's done. He's a good-looking kind and he's used that. [The team digresses for several exchanges about the patient's legal status. The patient had indicated that he believed his rights to due process had been violated. The social worker returns the team's focus to the patient's psychiatric problems by drawing a "negative" inference on how the patient says he's going to avoid his sentence.]

(166)    *Social Worker*: That's what was beginning to come when he said if he did it then my rights have been violated and so forth.... I don't think he really believes that he's going to face the sentence.

(167)    *Psychiatrist*: Yes, but he wants high school.

(168)    *Social Worker*: It's something to prove.

(169)    *Psychologist*: It looks good. That's all he wants it for.

(170)    *Social Worker*: You're saying he's psychopathic.

(171)    *Psychologist*: Yeah. Well, he got age in his.... I don't know if he has age in his favor or not. I'm not too sure. I kind of tend to think the other way. When they get into their late thirties, then they have age in their favor when they're psychopathic. [Several lines later members finalized their diagnostic theorizing.]

(177)   *Psychologist*: I think this guy is a classic sociopath. [The psychologist and psychiatrist continue this line of reasoning for several exchanges, pointing out how the patient is "really" not in touch with his own hostilities (lines 177-179), before the psychiatrist asks whether the team wants to "call him a psychopathic offender."]

(180)   *Psychiatrist*: . . .Do we want to call him a psychopathic offender?

(181)   *Psychologist*: I don't mind. I see this guy as a psychopath.

(182)   *Psychiatrist*: He's smooth. He's got connections.

(183)   *Psychologist*: He's smarter than the other guy, too.

(184)   *Psychiatrist*: Yeah, he's smart. He knows what to say.

In the preceding excerpt, traits that are commonly viewed in positive terms are transformed into retrospective indicators of psychopathy. Good looks (line 158), youthfulness (line 171), and the desire to finish school (line 169) are all viewed accordingly. In some other setting these traits may have been viewed as assets. Yet, having decided that the patient was a psychopath, the team selectively interprets each item as additional grounds for justifying the correctness of its theoretical inferences. Notice, for instance, that in the following excerpt a patient's good looks are used in an entirely different manner. Prior to the excerpted sequence, the psychiatrist has announced his decision that the patient is neither mentally ill nor dangerous. The psychologist is less sure. He has cited several "nonverbal" signals of the patient's "aggressive homosexuality" to justify his theory that the patient has problems in this area and may present problems for others. In the sequence presented below, the psychiatrist retrospectively buttresses his own conclusion by making inferences about the patient's physical attractiveness.

Excerpt 9-2. From Patient Review 71, Team J

(426)   *Psychiatrist*: Whether he's sexually homosexual or heterosexual isn't a whole bit difference in the ballgame. Because at least if he is homosexual he's not predatory. He certainly is a guy who engages in voluntary homosexual acts.

(427)   *Psychologist*: Well, I wonder if he might be . . . uh. . . . Well, but, uh. . . .

(428)   *Psychiatrist*: He's a good-looking guy. I think he could get homosexual partners if he wants 'em.

The employment of justificatory logic enabled review team members to recognize and solidify the "factual" basis of their decisions. By this logic, members were able to more clearly "see" a patient's past and more confidently predict his or her future. Through it they displayed for themselves and each other the "factual" basis for their decisions about an individual's psychiatric reality. In addition to selectively supporting such decisions, the retrospective logic of justification was also used to elaborate members' theorizing and to neutralize, transform, or modify the impact of potentially contradictory information. Each of these uses shall be considered in turn.

*Elaboration of Theorizing*

Rather than simply confirming previously arrived-at decisions, postinterview discussions typically expand theorizing in progress. The effect of such elaboration resembles a snowballing of observed symptoms. Many of a patient's verbal statements and nonverbal behaviors became retrospectively viewed as indicators of the expansive nature of his or her pathology. This process of elaboration is illustrated in the following excerpts. In the first, an "inappropriate look" documents the "fact" a patient is "sick as hell." In the second, a "homosexual gesture" observed by a psychologist is taken as evidence that this is the patient's basic problem. In the third, a patient's hope to continue his education is considered a sure sign of his inferiority complex. In the final excerpt, a patient's lack of insight into why he did not get a particular job was retrospectively interpreted as evidence that he was probably manifesting overt schizophrenic symptoms. Each of these excerpts exemplifies the power of a retrospective logic of justification in elaborating theories about psychiatric reality.

Excerpt 9-3. From Patient Review 50, Team B

(In receiving this patient's record the team noted reports of hallucinations and delusions. They suggested at that time the patient was "probably mentally ill" [line 26]. This excerpted exchange occurs shortly after the patient left the room. According to the observer, the patient in question had looked at the person asking him a question until the question was complete. In responding, however, he would look at the floor, look away at the wall, or look at the observer. At the same time, it should be noted that two of the team members were also observed as looking away or looking at their hands during much of the interview. Unlike these members, however, the patient was said to have a glossy-eyed look, which both the members and the observer attributed to the likely impact of medication. What exactly members literally saw in the patient's nonverbal self-presentation is unclear. The interpretation is not. They saw mental illness. Notice, moreover, how the social worker's statement that "I was beginning to have a sense of something" is glossed over, or let pass, as a valid observation. It is unlikely that members would have allowed the patient the free use of such "loose" inferential talk.)

(355)   *Social Worker*: I sensed that he was. . . . He left the room about five minutes ago. His look changed when you asked him [tape unclear]. Just a few minutes, maybe a minute or two before that, I was beginning to sense that there was something. He was having some kind of thoughts in his head that were unrelated to being here.

(356)   *Psychologist*: Yeah.

(357)   *Psychiatrist*: He's had a lot of thoughts in his head. I have a feeling that this man's still sick as hell.

Excerpt 9-4. From Patient Review 71, team J

(In this excerpt the psychologist elaborates his theorizing about a patient's problem with homosexuality by retrospectively interpreting a "rather long look" that the patient was said to have given the male observer. According to the observer the look was more indicative of interest in what the sociology graduate student was writing down in his notebook. Yet, according to the psychologist, this glance doesn't mean "anything much more than what we all suspect." The so-called long look of homosexual interest suggested to the clinician a "certain lack of control." This retrospective inference was taken at face value by the team. Again, it is hard to imagine the same clinicians letting such a statement pass as "valid reality testing," if it was made by a patient, instead of a clinician.)

(386)   *Psychologist*: Uh, one thing . . . I'm bothered by is his inability to remember all these things that he has been, or his inability to admit remembering. These things that he's done in the past are associated with homosexuality, and, uh, just. . . .

(387)   *Psychiatrist*: An arbitrary enough homosexual. . . .

(388)   *Psychologist*: I guess he's afraid that we'll decide against him, because he's, uh, homosexual. He feels some persecution about being, uh, judged a homosexual. And, uh, when he was talking about who he was attracted to, uh, I forgot the question that preceded it, whether or not you asked if he was a homosexual or what, I noticed he gave a rather long look to our observer here, and, uh, I don't think that means anything much more than what we all suspect.

(389)   *Psychiatrist*: Yeah.

(390)   *Psychologist*: But, uh, I think it suggests a certain, uh, lack of control, perhaps, uh, in that, uh, or lack of judgment. If he was trying to cover his homosexuality, which he seemed to be doing, he couldn't really disguise it.

Excerpt 9-5. From Patient Review 160, Team H

(The team is retrospectively reconstructing the patient's interview responses in light of their decision that he has an "inferiority complex." His desire to attend college is used to expand the team's theorizing about the patient's psychiatric reality.)

(826)   *Psychiatrist*: He is satisfied with a job of a grease monkey in a gas station so he can have two bucks per hour. And then when the sister comes into the picture, her parents send her to college, he wants to go to college.

(827)   *Psychologist*: Mmmm.

(828)   *Psychiatrist*: Feelings of inferiority. Not good at all as he quoted himself. And yet because he would like to measure up, it's a fantasy about going to school.

Excerpt 9-6. From Patient Review 50, Team B

(This team has already announced its theory that the patient is mentally ill. During the interview, the patient, a former social worker, was asked why he felt he did not get a job for which he interviewed. The patient did not know but felt that maybe it had something to do with the fact that he was inappropriately dressed in a striped jacket. The team here uses these comments by the patient in order to "see" how others saw him in the past. As the psychologist remarks, expanding the grounds for the team's present theorizing, "He was probably pretty deep into his schizophrenia and the other guy say it." This inference is rooted in the psychologist's retrospective logic alone.)

(365)    *Psychologist*: His insight was pretty good except that he'll never understand why he didn't get that job.

(366)    *Psychiatrist*: Striped shirt.

(367)    *Psychologist*: Striped shirt and jacket. That's the only reason he was rejected for the job, I guess.

(368)    *Social Worker*: We don't know how he behaved. You know, if he was afraid or whatever, he was.

(369)    *Psychologist*: Oh, well, he was probably pretty deep into his schizophrenia and the other guy saw it, whether he recognized it or not.


*Neutralizing, Transforming, or Modifying*
*"Contradictory" Information*

In the process of gathering data on patients, members occasionally uncovered information which potentially contradicted the direction of their previous theorizing. Members' typical response to this situation was to gloss over the potentially contradictory information in favor of getting the whole picture on a patient. This glossing took two forms. The most common was that of "passing-over." In this form possibly problematic information passed literally as unnoticed, unattended to, or unheard. Sometimes passing-over was not successful. One or more team members would raise the issue of potentially problematic information in the postinterview discussion. This led to efforts at a second form of glossing—"smoothing-over." This second glossing practice was a verbal one. It involved conversational displays of the essential irrelevancy of a piece of possibly contradictory information. The importance of this "new" information was minimized. Team members were asked to look beyond this irrelevant "fact" to grasp the whole picture of a patient's problems.

An example of glossing by "passing-over" involves a case in which members pushed the theory that a patient could probably never maintain meaningful relationships with the opposite sex. The patient, however, described involvement in a relatively long-term relationship. This response was never followed up during interviewing or during the postinterview discussion. The team passed over this information without allowing it to alter the whole picture that they were theoretically assembling.

Glossing by "smoothing-over" required greater work. This neutralization technique is exemplified in the following excerpt. During the diagnostic interview the patient raised certain doubts about the validity of his conviction. Members had been theorizing about the patient as a psychopathic individual. In accordance with this theorizing, the questions about the legality of commitment could be seen as just another attempt to manipulate. For the most part that is how the patient is heard. The team's psychologist, however, is not totally sure. Although he states that "I don't think he's innocent," the sense of possible contradiction still remains. According to the psychologist, "If he didn't commit these offenses, he doesn't need the treatment" (line 417). In a facinating display of retrospective logic, the other members neutralize the impact of this reasoning and justify their original theorizing. They can see that the patient is a psychopath whether or not he committed this specific crime (line 418). Reasoning backwards (even circuitously), the social worker suggests, "And he's in the psychopathic treatment unit, so the guilt has already been determined" (line 420). What the psychologist needs to do is ignore the irrelevant question about actual guilt and attend to the larger issue of the patient's obvious psychopathy. This the psychologist does (line 423) and the potential contradiction is smoothed over.

Excerpt 9-7. From Patient Review 330, Team J

(411)    *Psychologist*: I don't think he's innocent. . . . I don't expect he's innocent.

(412)    *Psychiatrist*: Well, that's not up to us to determine.

(413)    *Social Worker*: No, that doesn't really. . . . It's not our. . . .

(414)    *Psychiatrist*: This issue is, does he need the specific custody—yes, he goes.

(415)    *Psychologist*: Well, it is, though . . . relevant.

(416)    *Psychiatrist*: The treatment would be nice but . . . [psychiatrist and social worker both laugh].

(417)    *Psychologist*: If he didn't commit these offenses, he doesn't need the treatment.

(418)    *Social Worker*: Well, he's a psychopathic offender whether he committed these offenses or not. If you were talking to him and you never knew that he had these, these particular troubles, you'd still come to the conclusion, know he was a psychopathic offender.

(419)    *Psychologist*: Oh, yeah.

(420)    *Social Worker*: And he's in the psychopathic treatment unit, so the guilt has already been determined.

(421)  *Psychiatrist*: Do we agree with the diagnosis—that he ought to stay in custody? He needs the special setting.

(422)  *Social Worker*: He continues to need the care, custody, and treatment of this. . . .

(423)  *Psychologist*: Yeah. Good wording.

The glossing techniques of "passing-over" and "smoothing-over" are the ordinary means through which members neutralize potentially contradictory information. In some cases, however, these techniques are not allowed to work. Glossing is not permitted. In such cases, members are confronted with the resistance of a patient or some other member(s) that forcefully calls attention to a bit of contradictory information. When this occurs, members are presented with a dilemma. Should they defend previous theorizing or should they modify that theorizing in light of the "new" information? How members solve this dilemma appeared related to their perceptions of the mode in which patients presented themselves. In discussing this matter, we shall draw upon the distinctions among modes of patient self-presentation outlined in the previous chapter.

Members' solutions to the problem of unglossed contradictory information can be summarized in terms of two rules or propositions. The first states: *If members had previously theorized about a patient's problems in a particular fashion, and then the patient was perceived to be in the "denying" mode, the introduction of contradictory evidence will be transformed so as to support the idea of denial.* The second rule states: *If the patient was perceived in the "admitting" mode, the introduction of contradictory evidence will lead to certain retrospective adjustments in theorizing.* These adjustments erase the contradiction, as well as preserve the expertness of the theorizer.[1]

The use of the first rule (transforming contradictory information into evidence supporting "denial") is illustrated in the following excerpt. Here the patient is again said not to have the ability to enter into a committed relationship with others. Yet, the patient has expressed a desire to get married shortly after his release. More importantly, he pressed his point. He resisted efforts to gloss over this contradictory information by being quite emphatic about how realistic he "really" was about his marriage plans. He stated that he would be sure that he and the woman he married were compatible before marriage and talked about "working out problems" and even consulting a marriage counselor should tensions arise during the marriage. The psychiatric professionals, having theorized about the patient's lack of commitment to relationships, were faced with the dilemma of having previous theorizing jeopardized by new information. The solution to the challenge is displayed below. The contradiction is removed by transforming the patient's statements into additional evidence for what the clinician knew all along—that the patient only uses others to meet his own needs. The only reason he wanted to get married is "to be taken care of."

Excerpt 9-7. From Patient Review 441, Team D

(The social worker opens the postinterview discussion by initiating the following sequence.)

(385)    *Social Worker*: He sure wants to be taken care of.

(386)    *Psychiatrist*: Unfortunately.

(387)    *Psychologist*: Oh, I don't know.

(388)    *Social Worker*: To me, he wants to be taken care of. He keeps saying he wants a woman to keep him in line. He wants people to keep bad friends away from him. Uh, he's really not aware that he needs to do it himself.

The social worker, in the previous excerpt, was able to transform potentially positive information into actually negative information. This was done without perceiving any contradictions in the logic being employed. The patient was, after all, viewed not only as having problems but as denying having problems. Hence, in retrospect, it is easy to justify a theoretical understanding of how the patient failed to appreciate his own problems with wanting a marriage relationship "just to be taken care of." Once again, we observe the power of a retrospective logic of justification. However, if the patient is viewed as having problems but not denying them, the introjection of "new," contradictory information presents a different problem. If members accept the new information at face value, past theorizing would be open to question. The clinician's theorizing abilities would become circumspect.

The invocation of the second rule (adjusting one's theorizing while preserving the expertness of the theorizer) is a way out of the above dilemma. Having defined the patient as both having certain problems and being in the "admitting" mode, members retrospectively invent or "discover" facts extrnal to the review process which explain why members were partially misled in formulating their theories about a patient. The key element in this process is that the newly formulated "fact" alleviates members' responsibility for having theorized incorrectly. This new "fact" is presented as something which members could not have been aware of earlier. By retrospectively recognizing this "fact" members are spared the responsibility of having been wrong. This "fact" allows members to modify their original theorizing without jeopardizing their situated identity as an expert diagnostician.

The following excerpt represents an example of the use of retrospective justificatory logic in formulating face-saving new "facts." Before interviewing the patient in question, review of the record led to theorizing about him as a "schizey kind of a guy" with a mental deficiency. His crime was to have sexually molested a nine-year-old girl. During the interview, however, the patient satisfied team members by admitting his problem with sex, indicated that he had previously sought help voluntarily, and, if released, intended to do so again. He admitted the event for which he was charged, but explained it involved no coercive violence and was associated with much anxiety he was experiencing at the time. His coherence, admitted mode, remorse, and recognition of the consequences of his behavior all operated to contradict theorizing about him as "schizey" and mentally retarded. Had the team been wrong about these issues?

In the case being discussed, members modified their theorizing. They shifted to see the patient as "functioning adequately" rather than "schizey," and intelligent rather than retarded. Yet. making this modification. they discovered another "fact" that allowed them to shift interpretations without questioning the basis for their previous formulations. According to their modified reasoning, the reports they read (and from which they constructed their excessively negative theories about the patient) were the products of small-town, conservative biases. It was these reports that distorted the "real" facts of this case. Their own theorizing was not at fault. Note the deployment of this type of justificatory logic in the following postinterview discussion.

Excerpt 9-8. From Patient Review 424, Team B

(262) *Psychiatrist*: They must, if they're from small communities . . . the judge is afraid to . . . uh, there's votes involved.

(263) *Psychologist*: That is the point. [Name of place] is an awfully conservative county. Ultraconservative. That was a big, bad sex charge . . . evil, evil person. The things he did miss [in testing] were from anxiety and he still showed enough ability to abstract. . . . The proverbs—no, but the other abstractions—he did OK.

(264) *Psychiatrist*: Oh, give him another ten minutes and he would. . . .

(265) *Psychologist*: Yeah. If you could give him a little more permission and he could relax a little bit more, I know.

(266) *Psychiatrist*: I don't think he's at all retarded. I think he's of normal intelligence.

(267) *Psychologist*: Oh, no. He's not. This is what I thought we were going on [the previous record]—borderline mentally retarded.

(268) *Psychiatrist*: So did I. About the only note I have is not mentally retarded. I certainly agree with that—not mentally ill. Personality problem, but not mentally ill. Not mentally retarded. Not psychopathic offender.

Note that in the above excerpt once the retrospectively modified theory becomes the operative theory, members proceed to gloss over any further contradictions (for example, not doing well on the proverbs test). Retrospectively, members know and justify the "fact" that if they had "given him another ten minutes" he would have done well (line 264). Through this justificatory logic, members once again solidify their modified theory.

*The Logic of Reconciliation*

Through a logic of justification, members finalize the substance of psychiatric theorizing. Through a logic of reconciliation members show that this substance was discovered objectively and collectively. By it, members avoid the impression of divergence between their discoveries and those of other members. The public presentation of such divergence is threatening to members' presentations of themselves as expert diagnosticians. Overt displays of essentially different theorizing jeopardize the objective "fact" of a patient's psychiatric problems. If equally expert clinicians come to contradictory conclusions about the same patient, given cotemporal access to the same data, it could be reasonably argued that psychiatric problems are simply a subjective construct of the labeler. Thus, through a use of reconciliatory logic, members attend to and make efforts to reconcile possible differences in and among theoretical accounts of a patient's problems.

The use of reconciliatory logic has great practical significance in finalizing theories about patients. It guides theorizing in the direction of that with which all members are likely to agree. In general, that which does not show the promise of being collectively adopted is not perceived as being an adequate theoretical account. This is the power of a logic of reconciliation—the gatekeeping power of allowing certain accounts to pass as valid or objective, simply because they can be shared.

Like the logic of justification, members' logic of reconciliation displays certain rules which guide its use. These rules are summarized in a series of propositions. The first two of these propositions are quite general. The others function as modifiers or qualifiers of these very broad rules. The first proposition states: *If it is not perceived that members have already collectively announced a particular line of theorizing, members will begin the postinterview discussion with tentative (or suggestive) displays of their own theorizing.*

The formulation and public announcement of theories in tentative terms allow members to "feel out" the reactions of others without committing themselves to a definitive line of reasoning. Members' early statements suggest what they are thinking, but do not hold them accountable for having firmly defined a patient's psychiatric reality. If others respond supportively, tentativeness is abandoned and the theory is publicly stated in so many words. If others respond nonsupportively, members invoke a second rule of reconciliatory logic. In propositional form, this rule states: *If, in tentatively announcing their theorizing, members encounter the resistance of other members, they will modify or reformulate their thinking in accordance with that of the others.*

When members reformulate tentative theoretical offerings they ordinarily manage their conversation so as to suggest: "Yes, I agree with your disagreement, and in fact, that's what I was really suggesting all along anyway." This process of tentative formulation and reformulation is illustrated in the following excerpts.

Excerpt 9-9. From Patient Review 160, Team H

(This sequence occurs shortly after the patient leaves the room. The psychologist seems to offer a tentative formulation of the patient as nonretarded. In response to the psychiatrist's nonsupportive statements this offering is reaffirmed in terms of "it would be easier if he were more severely retarded." Thus is the appearance of reconciliation negotiated. The patient will be classified as definitely retarded.)

(811)    *Psychologist*: Mmm, he's a tough one.

(812)    *Psychiatrist*: I'm, uh.

(813)    *Psychologist*: He's too bright to be retarded, or at least it seems.

(814)    *Psychiatrist*: There are certain deficiency of intelligence.

(815)    *Psychologist*: Yeah. There's certainly a deficiency, only, um, it would be easier. . . . It seems as though it would be easier if he were more severely retarded.

In the preceding excerpt, the use of reconciliatory logic shifts members toward a more negative clinical judgment about a patient. In the following excerpt, the reverse occurs. In both cases, however, it is the attempt to reconcile which leads to the reformulation of a tentative theoretical offering. In this next excerpt, the social worker and psychologist begin to offer formulations which suggest that the patient is a psychopath (lines 399-400). When the psychiatrist disagrees with this line of theorizing (line 401), the members redefine their positions (lines 402-406) and display the "fact" that there was never any clinical disagreement in the first place. What may have appeared to be a disagreement really reflected a conflict in legal and psychiatric definitions, rather than a "real" difference among members. This reformulation both reconciles the expert opinions and provides an account for why the opinions temporarily appeared to be at variance. By line (421), the social worder and psychologist have moved together with the psychiatrist and away from their original theorizing. The patient, who was once tentatively called a psychopath, is finally theorized as neither psychopathic nor needing the confinement of Lima State Hospital.

Excerpt 9-10. From Patient Review 441, Team D

(399)    *Social Worker*: I guess he's a psychopathic offender, uh, gross immaturity, impulsive behavior.

(400)    *Psychologist*: He was concerned again more about his record and being caught.

(401)   *Psychiatrist*: I don't think he necessarily fits the . . . definition of a psychopathic offender.

(402)   *Psychologist*: No, he's not like the other, the first patient.

(403)   *Social Worker*: No, you mean in terms of impulsivity?

(404)   *Psychologist*: Well, there's more realistic hope or planning.

(405)   *Social Worker*: Yeah.

(406)   *Psychologist*: And there's more intelligence.

(407)   *Psychiatrist*: Yeah, there isn't the, it's almost the uncertainty that, uh, let's say I do, I don't know what's going to happen to a guy, the courts decide . . . the law says this. . . .

(408)   *Social Worker*: See, that's the trouble with that Ascherman Law.

(409)   *Psychologist*: Right.

(410)   *Social Worker*: He slips through the cracks onto it. No, we could say no, we don't believe he's an Ascherman case, although that wouldn't change his sentence.

(411)   *Psychiatrist*: No, see, that's the problem, too. We have a split here; well, is he a psychopathic offender in the psychiatric-psychological sense, is a little different than [*sic*] it is in the legal sense?

(412)   *Social Worker*: Yeah.

(413)   *Psychiatrist*: And that's all we're talking about. Sure, the law has to do what it says it has to do, but this guy's not helpless. He does have some insight, he has some expectations, and he has a fifty-fifty, as he says, chance of maybe getting probation. I think there's more drive toward, uh, how do I say.

(414)   *Psychologist*: There's less. . . .

(415)   *Psychiatrist*: Yeah, less antisocial . . . kinds of behavior.

(416)   *Psychologist*: Right.

(417)   *Social Worker*: I think we could simply avoid the psychopathic offender bit and not even say he's recovered or not, just go on and say he doesn't need care, custody, etc.

(418)   *Psychiatrist*: He's reached maximum benefit at Lima, those are his own words and I think our, at least my, feeling that he has. He's become chairman of something or other and he's gone along with it and so what is there, do you repeat it every year?

(419)   *Psychologist*: Right.

(420)   *Social Worker*: Yeah [pause].

(421)   *Psychiatrist*: . . . He doesn't need the maximum care and custody of this, but that doesn't say that we might be condemning him to some place worse. If some of the tales. . . .

(422)  *Psychologist*: Yeah, right. If he's to ever get out, he's got to get out of here first.

I have so far suggested that a logic of reconciliation guides members to make tentative statements of their theoretical positions and then to reformulate these positions if they encounter the resistance of others. These rules appear to be operative under two important conditions. First, members must perceive themselves to be dependent on the corroborative feedback of others to inform them of the essential accuracy of their theorizing. In the preceding excerpts, members' dependence on certain other members for corroboration in diagnosing "mental retardation" and "psychopathy" was a key element in their reformulation of tentative offerings. Second, members must not be so committed to particular lines of theorizing that they firmly announce and defend these theories. This can occur for a variety of reasons (for example, personal identification with a patient, professional investment in a particular diagnostic theme, the desire to "save face" or exert one's power as an expert). Regardless of the reason, a definite commitment to one line of theorizing alters the guidelines for the use of reconciliatory logic. So does the perceived lack of dependency on the collective corroboration of others. Rules which guide the use of reconciliatory logic under these conditions are outlined below.

Two additional rules guide members in conditions where corroboration is not depended upon. The basis for these rules arises in members' negotiations over power and status. These negotiations will be discussed later in this chapter. It is sufficient, at this time, simply to state what these rules are. The first states: *If one member is perceived as being more powerful than others, this member is allowed to firmly formulate and announce theories about patients, regardless of the resistance of others.*[2] In this situation, the less powerful persons would, by definition, be more dependent on the corroboration of the more powerful person, than she or he would be on them. This, of course, was the case in the two previous excerpts. It was the psychologists and social worker who shifted their tentative theorizing in the direction of the firmly stated positions of the psychiatrists. This is not to say that psychiatrists are always perceived as being more powerful. How exactly power is negotiated and claimed as a resource in practical theorizing is a topic we shall address later. What is important here is simply that perceived power imbalances make a difference in the use of reconciliatory logic.

A second rule qualifying the use of reconciliatory logic involved members who are interactionally stripped of their status as expert professionals. Again, this process of status degradation will be examined later. For the present, let us simply state: *If one member is no longer afforded the status of being an expert professional, other members need not consider this person's resistance in formulating and announcing theories about patients.* Members do not, in other words, have to reconcile their thinking with another member who is not perceived as a competent diagnostician. The "nonexpert's" thinking will be perceived as "off the wall" or "out of touch" with the real facts of a case. It will not have to be attended to in a reconciliatory fashion. As documented in the following excerpts, once a member has been situationally identified as a "nonexpert," her or his input can be overtly disagreed with, without jeopardizing the "objective" quality of members' general theorizing. In this case, there is no perceived conflict in expert opinions. The nonexpert's opinions are treated (depending on the evaluative context) as those of a "student" (who simply does not know as much), or as those of a "nuisance" (who keeps sidetracking serious diagnostic discussion). In the following excerpt the input of one member is afforded more "nuisance" than "expert" status.

Excerpt 9-11. From Patient Review 440, Team D

(It has just been suggested that the patient "definitely has a problem relating with females." The psychiatrist attempted to neutralize this negative inference by stating, "Don't we all." The social worker, however, decides to press this line of theorizing about the patient's sex problems. The patient's reaction to the observer is used as a document for this theorizing. This social worker, however, has been treated in the past as making "off-the-wall," unlikely, and unprofessional inferences. In the following sequence, the psychiatrist treats him as a "nonexpert" about the diagnostic matters at hand. By showing the social worker to be once again working in an "incorrect" framework, the psychiatrist erases the need to reconcile two expert but contradictory opinions.)

(394)   *Social Worker*: Some are better [at dealing with females] than others, though. [The social worker then directs comments to the female observer.] I was, by the way, trying to signal you to stop your foot-moving.

(395)   *Observer*: My foot moving? Oh.

(396)   *Social Worker*: Are you nervous? [Again, this is directed to the observer.]

(397)   *Psychiatrist*: Why? Why would you want to stop her foot from moving?

(398)   *Social Worker*: Well, I thought it might distract the patient.

(399)   *Psychiatrist*: Well, he probably thought it was cute.

(400)   *Social Worker*: Well, it's cute, but, uh. . . .

(401)   *Psychiatrist*: Well, the fact is that he kept on and it didn't distract him.

(402)   *Social Worker*: Yeah.

A final rule which qualifies the use of reconciliatory logic involves situations in which members show definite commitment to different lines of theorizing. In such situations members seek to reconcile their differences without relinquishing the basis for their respective theories. This is accomplished by reframing questions in such a way that the theorizing appears complementary rather than contradictory. In propositional form: *If members display commitment to essentially different lines of theorizing, they will reframe questions about psychiatric reality so as to underscore the complementary nature of theorizing.*

The reframing practices through which members reconcile articulated differences in theorizing ordinarily involve several steps. The first is for members to deflect attention away from differences and provide time to display a sense that they are pursuing the same goal in basically the same way. Deflection, in other words, provides an opportunity to "cool out" opposition and emphasize solidarity. Otherwise, members are likely to find themselves conversationally locked into a debatelike conflict in theorizing. In deflecting attention away from differences members frequently "derail" the current topic by introducing an extraneous and nonproblematic issue for consideration. This deflection through derailing is illustrated in the following excerpts.

In the first excerpt a psychiatrist and psychologist display differences in whether or not a particular patient should be classified as a sociopath. The psychiatrist, stressing the patient's long criminal history, says yes. The psychologist, when comparing "this guy" to the man the team saw previously ("a real sociopath"), thinks not. Although he would accept a secondary diagnosis as an "antisocial personality," he feels that the real problem is an "inadequate personality" or "mood disorder" (line 120). The psychiatrist, on the other hand, stresses that both "this guy" and "the other guy" show the same denial behaviors which are typical of the sociopath (line 121). In response, the psychologist appears to claim that in contrast to the other guy "who has been in jail so much that it must have been him" (line 124), this guy's story (which the psychiatrist sees as denial) has a "flavor of belief" (122). Thus, point for point, members seem to reemphasize rather than resolve their differences. When this occurs the social worker appears to assume a mediational role. This member deflects the apparent conflict by derailing the topic (line 126). The members temporarily digress from their disagreements, referring themselves instead to the confusing nature of "the incident" in general.

Excerpt 9-12. From Patient Review 421, Team B

(The psychologist begins this excerpted sequence by stating that he does not think the patient is a sociopath. He then proceeds to contrast this patient with the last patient reviewed by the team.)

(120)   *Psychologist*: The other guy we saw before I thought was. This is a mere history of repeated legal or social offenses. It's not sufficient to justify this designation. This guy has that. He has the repeated offenses. But I don't see this guy as a sociopath. Well, yeah, that's hard to argue. But I see him, the secondary diagnosis in my book would be antisocial personality. First, I see this guy as an inadequate personality. Some kind of mood disorder or whatever.

(121)   *Psychiatrist*: See. Both of these [this man and the previous man] are the typical denial. . . .

(122)  *Psychologist*: Just a flavor of belief for that, though [for this man's story].

(123)  *Psychiatrist*: Yeah.

(124)  *Psychologist*: This guy's got the reputation of being the bad guy. That guy's been in jail so much that it must have been him. I'm not saying he's. . . .

(125)  *Psychiatrist*: I don't think. . . .

(126)  *Social Worker*: This whole incident. I'm really confused in terms of, I was trying to read and there are so many, there are five counts, for example.

In the second excerpt a social worker and psychologist have attempted to document a picture of the patient as a manipulator. The psychiatrist has suggested that what they call manipulation might reflect a "normal" desire to put one's foot forward. Rather than continue the debate, the social worker derails the conversation to a more neutral topic (lines 413-415).

Excerpt 9-13. From Patient Review 442, Team D

(410)  *Psychiatrist*: I didn't think he was lying. I think he was putting his best foot forward, but what else is he going to do?

(411)  *Social Worker*: Right. Manipulation is the name of the game. That's what's being done. . . .

(412)  *Psychiatrist*: Well, I don't know if that's manipulating. I wouldn't call it that. I don't know what they mean by manipulating, unless, oh, what will I say? He doesn't want ceramics. It's basically nothing to do with any good here. So, he doesn't want this program or that program and he's impatient to get to vocational training at [name of prison]. Uh, this kind of quality has a [logic element] to his behavior rather than the demand for immediate satisfaction.

(413)  *Social Worker*: Uh, he's been here since July.

(414)  *Psychiatrist*: Right.

(415)  *Social Worker*: And, of course, here again is that question of whether to keep the guy here for the so-called program.

The derailing of conflict-directed conversation buys time, but it does not secure reconciliation. The movement from contradiction to complementation is facilitated by a second step, in which members begin to reemphasize all the things that they basically agree on. In the sequence considered in excerpt 9-12 the disagreeing members pause to emphasize that they both agree on the patient's need for treatment and that behaviorally the patient fits the legal definition of a psychopathic offender. In excerpt 9-13, members take time to display their agreements that the individual "certainly" acted like a psychopathic offender prior to coming to the hospital and that he had been in the hospital but a very short time (five months).

By itself, the refocusing on agreed-upon findings does not provide a final reconciliation between team members with different theories. What it does provide is a set of common "discoveries" from which to construct a new theory which incorporates, rather than contrasts, divergent theorizings. In light of this newly constructed theory, the old theories are allowed to pass as complementary instead of contradictory. The oneness of diagnostic expertise is preserved and the substance of a psychiatric decision is finalized.

The accomplishment of reconciliation through the invention of a new, more encompassing theory is illustrated by returning to the two "disagreeing sequences" examined above. In the first, the team discovers that "need for treatment" is a more salient issue than whether or not one technically calls the patient a psychopathic offender. When this theory is announced, the previous disagreements are retrospectively viewed as complementing each other. According to the team's psychiatrist, its members have arrived "at the same conclusion for different reasons." The psychologist is now satisfied with calling the patient a psychopathic offender as long as the final report notes that the patient suffers more from an inferiority complex and that he is not a standard psychopathic offender (line 170). If these conditions are met, disagreements fade to the background and team members produce for themselves and their audience a sense of essential agreement in the decision reached.

Excerpt 9-14. From Patient Review 421, Team B

(The psychologist has just expressed his agreement with the psychiatrist that the patient needs treatment and that behaviorally he has acted like a psychopathic offender, although "psychiatrically" he is more of an inadequate personality.)

(141) *Psychologist*: In order to keep him here we'd have to label him a psychopathic offender. Behaviorally he is.

(142) *Psychiatrist*: He's not psychotic. It's a character disorder.

(143) *Psychologist*: That's my problem, because I don't see him, well. . . .

(144) *Psychiatrist*: Well, despite what he's saying, he thinks he'd be better off in jail. If this guy is going to be incarcerated, I think his chances are a little bit better here.

(145) *Psychologist*: That's what I'm saying.

(146) *Psychiatrist*: I'm in favor of that.

(147) *Psychologist*: Whatever. He needs to be locked up, but, yet, treated or get treatment.

(The members continue to emphasize this line of "new" theorizing for several more exchanges. The psychiatrist then begins to formulate the final report, suggesting that the patient is a "psychopathic offender." The psychologist responds by reminding the psychiatrist to include data about the patient's inadequate personality in the report. This was the core of the psychologist's previous theorizing. When the psychiatrist agrees, the psychologist initiates the following summary comments.)

(170)   *Psychologist*: It's hard to argue that, in any case, that this guy is not a psychopathic offender. He's here. You almost have to call him. . . . You don't have to, but it would be hard to argue. He's not a standard psychopathic offender.

(171)   *Psychiatrist*: Are we agreed that. . . .

(172)   *Psychologist*: Yeah. I'm agreed with that.

Once members achieve complementary theorizing their guiding logic shifts from reconciliation to justification. This is evident in the last several lines of excerpt 9-13. The psychologist, who once refused to see the patient as a psychopathic offender, retrospectively reasons that "you almost have to call him" that (line 170). Clearly, this justified and reconciled reversal is evidence of the power of the two forms of logic guiding members substantive decision-making.

The same pattern of reconciliation and justification is evidenced in the final excerpt of this section. The psychiatrist who in excerpt 9-12 argued that it was reasonable (and not manipulative) for the patient not to participate in the hospital program has been reconciled to the "new" theory that the patient has not really been at the hospital long enough to find out if he can benefit from the program. Under this "new" theory, the psychiatrist's assessment of the patient's action as "reasonable" and the other members' assessment of these as "manipulative" blend as complementary rather than contradictory. Since he was new to the hospital and experiencing considerable stress, it is "reasonable" to see how he would try to get out (even manipulatively) before he ever really knew what the program had to offer. Having reconciled themselves to this complementary conclusion, members justify this decision in the following manner:

Excerpt 9-15. From Patient Review 422, Team B

(444)   *Psychologist*: He's been in here five months. So I don't know if he's really had a chance to see what he's going to do in the program here, versus the fourteen months. [The reference to fourteen months is the length of time that the previous patient had been institutionalized. This is another example of team's comparison of one patient with another.]

(445)   *Social Worker*: Yeah. That I could say. That fourteen months was maybe long enough.

(446)   *Psychologist*: But five isn't. I don't think.

(447)   *Psychiatrist*: OK, then he should stay here, due to the shortness of time and repetitions. . . .

(448)   *Social Worker*: Maybe we can put it that way. That he, uh, hasn't been here long enough to properly evaluate the results of the program here.

(449)   *Psychologist*: Because he's really not into much of it.

(450)   *Psychiatrist*: See, there may be a time, I don't know, when he sees, "Well, I'm not going anywhere," that he accepts it a little more. And then the staff can get a better evaluation, too, whether he is or isn't going to make it; one way or the other.


## Additional Characteristics of Psychiatric Decision-Making

In addition to the interplay between justificatory and reconciliatory logic, the substance of final theorizing about patients is contingent upon several other characteristic elements of psychiatric decision-making. Negotiations over status and power, anticipation of the consequences of making particular recommendations, and the use of individual theorizing about psychiatric troubles all impact directly upon final decisions.


## Negotiating Status and Power

The substantive formulation of final decisions was significantly affected by the ongoing negotiation of status and power. On most teams one member was deferred to by others as someone possessing a higher status as an expert. This higher expert status was indicated by several deference patterns. First, opinions of higher status members were sought more frequently than those of others. Second, the diagnostic opinions of higher status members were most often those toward which reconciliatory reformulations were directed. Third, the suggested diagnostic wordings of higher status members were most frequently written into teams' final reports. Moreover, once members were deferred to as persons with greater expertise, they could use this higher status as a (reflexive) resource through which to exert power in formulating the substance of a given psychiatric recommendation. In other words, they could use their higher expert status as a means to obtain the recommendation they wanted, even against the resistance of others.

In considering the influence of status and power on psychiatric decision-making, three questions emerge. Who are the higher status members? How is it that members become deferred to as persons of higher expert status? How is it that higher expert status, once attained, operates as a resource in the exertion of power?

In addressing the first question, it should be noted that psychiatrists were observed as clearly higher status experts on seven of eleven teams. On these teams, members deferred to psychiatrists' judgments, opinions, and predilections in all phases of the patient review process. On three other teams, psychiatrists were observed as being deferred to in the formulation of final decisions, but were not viewed as dominating all phases of the review process. On these teams the division of expert labor was such that each member was treated as an expert in different aspects of the decision-making task. Psychologists were generally treated as possessing considerable expertise in assessing emotional and intellectual functioning. Social workers were viewed as being expert in the area of legal knowledge. The expert opinions of psychologists and social workers were readily sought in these respective areas of specialization. The opinions of psychiatrists, however, were still deferred to in the final formulation of a diagnostic opinion. It was as if psychiatrists predominated in defining a team's logic of justification, while the expertise of other members was limited to the teams' logic of discovery. On only one team was another member (a psychologist) viewed as having greater diagnostic expertise than the psychiatrist.

The manner in which members defer to the expertise of one another will be exhibited in discussing how status operates as a resource in the exertion of power. For the present, let us turn to the question of how members become viewed as persons of differentially high expert status. Each member joined her or his review team, having the officially certified credentials of a psychiatric professional. Yet the attainment of high expert status was not something which came automatically or which could be taken for granted. It required that members, from the onset, present themselves in certain ways, come off in a particular fashion, and manage interactions with others in such a manner that they would be granted the status of expert professional in the eyes of their coworkers. The accomplishment of an identity as an expert, in other words, was a situated achievement which required considerable work.

The suggestion that expert status emerges in the interactional work of members does not imply that all members have equal resources in performing this work. In fact, members do not enter the arena of status negotiation on equal footing. The traditional preeminence of the psychiatrist in guiding the medical discovery of mental illness was well known to all members. It was also recognized that the psychiatrist and psychologist were likely to have had more years of professional training than the social worker. These were potential symbols of status deference which were unlikely to be neutralized by the official doctrine that all team members were to be considered as equals and that the so-called medical model would not necessarily dictate the style of the patient reviews. Nonetheless, potential symbols of status deference were abstract resources which awaited realization in concrete interactions between members. Psychiatrists were not automatically afforded higher status. If they were seen as more expert than other members, it was because they worked to achieve this differential evaluation. Most psychiatrists succeeded in doing exactly this. The following is a list of expert status attainment practices which members (particularly psychiatrists) employed to secure the achievement of higher status.

## 1. Displaying "Medical" Knowledge as Indispensable Expertise

This was a status attainment practice which psychiatrists alone could employ. What emerged in members' interactions with each other was the sense that, while psychiatrists knew quite a bit about what psychologists and social workers knew (about psychological testing or family dynamics, etc.) psychologists and social workers generally knew little about what psychiatrists, as physicians, knew. By displaying this disparity in mutual knowledge, psychiatrists were able to create and sustain the appearance of being indispensable experts. In general, psychiatrists made full use of their medical knowledge as a status resource. They frequently commented on the possible organicity of a patient's problems and explained the basis for any other physical symptoms or troubles the patient may have encountered. It was the topic of psychotropic medication, however, which psychiatrists most consistently used to show their indispensable expertise. Often psychiatrists would correct other members' mispronunciation of the names of certain medications and comment technically on side effects and expected physiological reactions. Hence, the topic of medication provided psychiatrists with the opportunity to display knowledge that others did not possess.

## 2. Displaying One's Professional Credentials

Another status attainment practice typically employed by psychiatrists was to "matter of factly" reveal that one has a long list of professional credentials to back up one's performance as an expert. It was common, for instance, to hear psychiatrists talk about how they had been the director of this center or testified in that court setting. As observed previously, psychiatrists appeared to have had the most previous contact with maximum-security patients. Yet past experience is useless as a status resource unless it is introduced as a topic in actual conversation. Members have not, after all, read each other's vitae. This fact was not overlooked by most psychiatrists who often displayed their credentials for others to see, hear, and be impressed by. The following excerpt represents an illustration of such a display.

Excerpt 9-16. From Patient Review 71, Team J

(The psychologist has just made the observation that the patient appears to be covering up a problem with homosexuality. The psychiatrist, in disagreeing, displays his superior expertise, by referring to two papers he has written and to his fourteen years of experience.)

(391)  *Psychiatrist*: Oh, I don't know. I think if he were really an active homosexual he wouldn't be at all uncomfortable about it. I think that, uh, first, I've spent about, you know, I've written those two papers on homosexuality and treated them for about fourteen years now. So, I don't. I think he's probably, if there's a homosexual component, it may be the flight from the obvious incestuous feelings he had with mother.

### 3. Displaying Demonstration of Specialized Psychiatric Knowledge

Another strategy of status attainment was to provide expositions of special knowledge on certain general psychiatric topics which other members had little knowledge of. Psychiatrists were observed providing such expositions in two fashions. The first entailed a lecturelike explanation of some theory of mental illness or aspect of psychiatric treatment. The second was to actually use the patient as an example of some topic of theoretical interest and thereby demonstrate something to other team members. These two styles of demonstrating specialized knowledge are illustrated in the following excerpts. In the first, a psychiatrist pauses to lecture his coworkers about the meaning of malingering, and as the psychiatrist spells out the name "G-a-n-s-e-r," the other members are almost cast into the role of students. In the second, the psychiatrist rises out of his chair, place his hands on a patient, and proceeds to treat this individual as an exhibit of certain physiological symptoms associated with a particular nervous-system disease.

Excerpt 9-17. From Patient Review 210, Team G

(121)   *Psychiatrist*: The question asked if he was malingering. Very often a person, uh, this happens in, this happens in, uh, persons incarcerated. That, uh, he might have committed an act but [we] don't have a good history as to what happened. But then, uh, he may, he may, he may pretend that he was ill at the time. And, uh, for sure, for that he may become ill. And then they're at getting the question then of trying to, well, uh, to, to maintain a front. He doesn't know, and soon becomes malingering. And every now and then he comes back to reality and they'd ask, and when he speaks to that, he's really not able to. He might even become very assaultive or very angry, which you can't do with . . . malingerers, or, uh. This happens when you speak of, uh, another syndrome, the Ganser syndrome. G-a-n-s-e-r, where the person unconsciously becomes disturbed. I mean, it's a protective device. Once he's out of a situation then he returns to normal, to normal . . . functioning. So, this has to do with—we're dealing with an individual who is a clear-cut schizophrenic and who's in need of treatment here.

Excerpt 9-18. From Patient Review 162, Team H

(365)   *Psychiatrist*: Do you have a special gait when you walk? Maybe you can demonstrate this to us, all right? Would you please get up, and without paying attention to us, walk to the door? All right, now come back. All right, now, since I have you in this position, put your feet together. Put your arms like this. And now close your eyes, close your eyes. All right. Oh, you are doing this very well. Now, open your eyes and we will do this. Lift up your arms in this position. All right, but you can put your feet down more comfortably, but straight out, and with closed eyes. But keep the eyes closed. OK, lift up your left arm as much as you can, and put it back to the same position it was before. And do the same with the right, now. And back to the same position. Now, do you

have difficulties to close your eyes? Close your eyes. Don't be afraid. Can you keep them closed? This is another very interesting symptom. Show this to them, because they do not see this too often, all right? Try to close completely. You have no reason to be afraid, we are friendly people. OK. Please sit down.

## 4. Displaying a Nonverbal Posture of Confidence and Control

This status-attainment practice involves a variety of nonverbal behaviors which display that one is relaxed, confident, and in control. These things may be indicated, for instance, in the manner in which one sits. Psychiatrists, who attained the deference of others, typically leaned back in their chairs, often stretching or putting their hands behind their heads. It was as if these members were claiming an easy familiarity with the hospital environment and setting. Other members were ordinarily described as more frequently leaning forward. Their postures were generally more intense or less relaxed.

The use of visual attentiveness also appeared to be a gesture involved in displaying status prerogatives. When a psychiatrist spoke, others generally positioned themselves (their posture and eyes) in the direction of the speaker. When psychiatrists reviewed or commented upon the patient's record, other members often took notes. Yet, when others were speaking, psychiatrists frequently looked away ponderously. When others reviewed the record, psychiatrists often appeared to occupy themselves with something elss (for example, leafing through the record). This is not to say that the psychiatrists were not listening. They often asked questions, though frequently without looking up or toward the other members. These gestures were not distributed evenly among team members. They are interpreted as gestural aspects of successfully managed status-attainment practices. These gestures let others know that one is comfortable with the work at hand and less dependent on others than others are on oneself.

## 5. Displaying Clinical Skills by Taking Charge of the Interview

During diagnostic interviews psychiatrists routinely displayed their expert status by taking charge during critical moments. When not questioning, they would typically sit in such a fashion as to not be directly facing the patient. However, when they decided that another member was not making her or himself clear to the patient or that the other member was pursuing an inappropriate line of questioning, they would gesturally and conversationally cut back into the interview. The psychiatrist would (like the experienced clinical instructor) take charge and attempt to guide the patient through any difficulties in the interview. This process of cutting into another's line of questioning is illustrated in the following excerpts. The psychiatrist displays a "teacherlike" mode of intervention as he shows disapproval of the manner in which the social worker has been asking "leading questions."

Excerpt 9-19. From Patient Review 442, Team D

(206) *Social Worker*: Everybody was boasting about getting arrested and thrown in jail and so on, or, if it was a stolen car?

(207) *Patient*: Mmmm, yes.

(208) *Psychiatrist*: Is that the way you felt or did he put some thoughts in your mind?

Psychiatrists also displayed the prerogative to simply "cut in" with other lines of questioning when they perceived that the other clinicians were getting nowhere. They also cut in to make explanatory comments like that depicted in the following interview. Each of these interventions served a substantive purpose. They also reinforced the idea that the psychiatrist was really the "expert in charge."

Excerpt 9-20. From Patient Review 162, Team H

(The patient has been talking about some neurological tests in which something like a "flashlight" was shone in his eyes. Notice how the psychiatrist "cuts in" to make things expertly clear.)

(467) *Patient*: That flashlight, and it felt like I was going back in the past, bringing all these things out.

(468) *Psychologist*: Uh-huh.

(469) *Patient*: And this bugged me, too. I didn't like that.

(470) *Psychologist*: Do you know why they gave you this flashlight?

(471) *Patient*: They, they thought that I had a brain, uh, something wrong with my mind.

(472) *Psychiatrist*: No, I will tell you. This is a photostimulation, that when one sees a flickering light, [a person] who has seizures can get under influence. An epileptic, when he drives a car on a sunny day on a street with trees coming from shade into light, is exposed to flickering stimulation. The same is on television that he watches and flickers and then, can have a convulsion. See, this was the purpose, the technician did this in order to find out if this can provoke a seizure, you know.

A final illustration of the way psychiatrists routinely take charge of an interview was by defining that point at which the interview would end. Often, they would ask the other members if they had any other questions. Sometimes (as in the following excerpt), they would simply cut into another member's questioning, thank the patient for coming, and thereby end the interview. This process of announcing the end of an interview was another vehicle psychiatrists used to display their expert status.

Excerpt 9-21. From Patient Review 363, Team L

(The social worker appears to be in the middle of a sequence of questions about the patient's relationship to his family. The psychiatrist simply cuts in to end the interview. Notice how this ending shifts into a beginning of the postinterview discussion. The psychiatrist very "untentatively" leads off with a rather definite picture of his diagnostic theorizing.)

(89) *Social Worker*: Have you heard from your wife or your children?

(90) *Patient*: No. Not al all since I've been up here. Just ended the relationship.

(91) *Psychiatrist*: Thank you very much for coming in to talk with us.

(92) *Patient*: They don't know what happens now?

(93) *Psychiatrist*: We understand you will be receiving a copy of our final recommendations very shortly. In a few days.

(94) *Patient*: Does this change their staffing procedure here now?

(95) *Psychiatrist*: No. There's no changing of staffing and no conflict or disagreement with staff, of course. This is just our recommendation as to whether we feel you're ready to leave here or wherever you should go from here, based on the law. And if you'll receive maximum benefit from being here, and do you still need to be here? This is the type of thing we're trying to find out.

(The patient leaves and the psychiatrist immediately begins his postinterview theorizing.)

I saw the depression. Then his wife started acting up, and he started depressing more. Then he had an accident and after the accident he lost—he lost everything—physically, mentally. He lost everything. Then he began drinking more and more.

In observing that psychiatrists displayed a general tendency to cut into and take charge of diagnostic interviews, I am not suggesting that they were in any way better clinicians than others. I am simply observing that they generally cut in and took over interview talk at times when the questioning became confused or strained, when they felt that an "expert" clarification was needed, and when they believed the interview should be terminated. Other members did not cut into psychiatrists' questioning in the same manner. The only set of cases in which other members "cut in" on the psychiatrists involved the one team in which the psychiatrist appeared to lack the deferential respect of others. However, in the two teams in which psychiatrists were observed to be influential, but not dominating, the types of interventions described here rarely took place.

*6. Displaying Oneself as Representing the Team*

Another device for claiming status was to present oneself as the team's representative to external agents (that is, the research observers, hospital and mental health officials, and the court). Psychiatrists had an advantage here. Perhaps because of traditional assumptions about their leadership role, they would ordinarily be approached by outside agents "as if" they were in charge. This was generally the case with the research observers who ordinarily attempted to identify themselves first to the team's psychiatrist. It was also the case with hospital personnel who, when speaking with a team, would ordinarily address its psychiatrist. This observation is also made by a psychologist in the following excerpt.

Excerpt 9-22. From Psychologist Interview

They [psychiatrists] were addressed by the officials whenever a question came up. They were addressed by the attendants or the team and everything funneled up to them from day one and hour one. So whether they themselves had—of course many of them had—set themselves up to be leaders, from time one the other people involved also collaborated in this type of thing because you just don't, the image is there, and you don't change.

To make full use of this device as an indicator of higher status, members had to actively claim the role of mediator between the team and outside agents. Most psychiatrists assumed this role. They were the persons who explained (or re-explained) to other members what the research observers really wanted and how the team would cooperate with them. They were the persons who claimed more extensive or greater knowledge about what the court and legal section wanted from teams. The exceptions to this were the two teams with a more equal division of labor and the team in which the psychiatrist did not "come off" as a person of higher status. On those teams, definitions of what external agents were about or what they wanted from teams were negotiated by all members. As mentioned previously, sometimes the social worker in the "more equal" teams was the person looked to as having greater legal knowledge of the technical requirements of the law and the court order.

On teams in which psychiatrists claimed expertise in interpreting what the court "really" meant, sometimes their claims were just that. Occasionally, their interpretations represented no particular "factual" correlation to the court order as it was written. For instance, when one team, which was reviewing a penal transfer, diagnosed the patient as a psychopath, the psychiatrist declared that they now had to consult the guidelines for "Ascherman" cases. He apparently had confused the clinical idea of psychopathy with the legal category of psychopathic offender. Yet, this confusion passed as "fact." The teams' clinical decisions were directed in terms of the legal definitions provided by this expert member.

Another example of a misfounded display of expert knowledge is excerpted below. The psychiatrist is interpreting for others the supposed role of the referee in reviewing members' decisions. Actually the court order makes no reference to a referee. As the psychologist attempts to point out, it is the "master" who is to oversee the case (line 638). The psychiatrist rejects or passes by this suggestion, although he later uses this same term (line 643). When the psychologist tries to claim prior knowledge of this topic (line 644), his statement is derailed by the psychiatrist, who jumps on the term "formally" and states, "No. There's no formality in the process" (line 646). Apparently what is important here is not that the psychiatrist can talk accurately, but that he can talk with the appearance of being very knowledgeable. From the reports of observers and members alike, the psychiatrist in this case was very successful in doing exactly that. As the transcript continues, we see evidence that he has persuaded the social worker of his knowledgeability. The social worker expresses agreement with the psychiatrist's definition of the situation (line 647). The psychologist whose interventions have been talked away finally defers to the psychiatrist's role as mediator. Rather than continuing the challenge the psychologist offers another question through which the psychiatrist can display further mediative knowledge.

Excerpt 9-23. From Patient Review 212, Team G

(The psychiatrist and psychologist have been exchanging comments on what happens if they say that a patient is "restored to reason." The psychiatrist then attempts to take charge of the discussion and display his knowledge of how the legal procedures work.)

(635)    *Psychiatrist*: The judge then would have to act, and only the judge can act. Right? This is how it works.

(636)    *Psychologist*: Mmm. Not only to stand the trial, or skip that part, to review what we say. . . .

(637)    *Psychiatrist*: Oh. Oh, that has to be done, but it's done differently. You have the uh, what you call 'em, the uh, the uh, the help. He has here a couple of case. . . .

(638)    *Psychologist*: The master.

(639)    *Psychiatrist*: No. Yeah, what'd they call him? They call him the. . . . The judge appoints . . . someone to hear a case.

(640)    *Social Worker*: You mean a public attendant or something.

(641)    *Psychiatrist*: No. What do yóu call a person. He's a judge. He's acting in place of the judge?

(642)    *Social Worker*: Referee?

(643)    *Psychiatrist*: Referee. See, this is under the referee. The referees coming in. This is the master that we were referring to.

(644)    *Psychologist*: Well, he's called formally. . . .

(645)    *Psychiatrist*: No. There's no formality. The referee is disposed and reports back to the judge. And the judge OKs it. And if the judge is not satisfied, he'll want to see him personally.

(646)    *Social Worker*: Personally. Yeah.

(647)    *Psychiatrist*: The referee has to have all these acted upon, what we say. . . .

(648)    *Psychologist*:[Well, the patient, then] how does he get out of [this] place, in case they follow our recommendation?

(649)    *Psychiatrist*: The patient? Well, we just say that, you just say that he's, that he's, uh, his psychosis is in remission with the use of medication. At this time he's [deserving] and placed in a less restrictive situation and geared toward gradual removal, I mean, uh, back into the community. So I mean, you know, you can list all the stuff he needs to be and jazz it up there.

## 7. Displaying Control over Others' Expert Identities

A central purpose-at-hand for all members was to establish identities as expert professionals.[3] The various status attainment strategies discussed to this point were employed primarily by psychiatrists to establish their own positions as the highest ranking expert. This does not mean that others could not also "come off" as experts, although perhaps as experts of lesser status. Others could establish expert identities but ordinarily were dependent on the prerogative of psychiatrists in doing so.

Most psychiatrists displayed a certain control over the granting of expert identities to others. This entailed letting other members know that psychiatrists, if they chose, could undermine others' efforts to appear as experts. In this sense, psychiatrists displayed the ability to punish others by withholding a valued reward—the establishment of an expert identity. On the other hand, psychiatrists also had to display the ability to reward. This rewarding of others was typically accomplished by concurring with their theorizing and thus allowing members to accomplish a sense of professional expertise.

The ability of a psychiatrist to punish other members by pointing out problems with their performance as experts is illustrated at several other places in this report. We have observed a psychiatrist reprimanding members for confusing theorizing with factual documentation (excerpt 7-12). We have also noted how psychiatrists may "cut into" others' interviewing and challenge the leading nature of their questioning (excerpt 9-20). In instances such as these, the psychiatrist displays subtle reminders of his power to give and take away another's identity as an expert. Certainly whenever the psychiatrist casts himself in a role resembling the clinical instructor he claims for himself the ability to distribute professional rewards and punishments (excerpt 9-17). One psychiatrist, who was particularly skilled in such displays, would routinely open postinterview discussions with invitations for the other team members to try their hand at theorizing. He would lead off with such statements as "OK, gang, prognostic formulation, dynamic formulation. Who will give it a try?"

Other techniques which display one's ability to grant or withhold expert identities included ignoring certain statements made by others while immediately challenging the tone or accuracy of other statements. These practices kept others' expert identities in question. Psychiatrists would let certain things pass as if they had not ever been said. Other things, which were not meant to be taken seriously, were picked up on and exposed as less-than-expert accounts. Psychiatrists, in other words, even exercised a certain control over when jokes would be allowed to be heard as jokes and when they would be treated as nuisancelike distractions from more serious matters at hand. So too would they offset the timing in others' presentation of information. Note in the following excerpt how the psychiatrist displays control over what information will be presented when. In doing so the psychiatrist reminds the team member that how one comes off as a professional depends on how the psychiatrist allows one to come off.

Excerpt 9-24. From Patient Review 211, Team G

(The social worker is attempting to present a set of rather elaborate notes on the patient's record. The psychiatrist interrupts the presentation.)

(7)   *Psychiatrist*: Where was that? Here or West Virginia?

(8)   *Social Worker*: This was here. I assume Hamilton County.

(9)   *Psychiatrist*: OK.

(10)   *Social Worker*: Yeah. Because he was returned there. OK.

(11)   *Psychiatrist*: Why was he admitted here this time?

(12)   *Social Worker*: Well, OK, let me. I was going to get to that later, but I do it slowly. [The social worker returns to a set of notes and begins a detailed description of the events leading to commitment. The psychiatrist interrupts in the "middle" of the social worker's presentation.]

(13)   *Psychiatrist*: There's one thing you haven't answered, though.

(14)   *Social Worker*: What's that?

(15)   *Psychiatrist*: Why was he sent originally in January of '74?

(16)   *Social Worker*: I'm trying to. I just told you. That wasn't his original. He was sent back as. . . .

(17)   *Psychiatrist*: I know. What was his original as opposed to. . . .

(18) *Social Worker*: Oh, the shooting, for murder second degree. That was in 1964.

(19) *Psychiatrist*: Yeah.

(20) *Social Worker*: And after being here ten years he had improved, so they. . . .

(21) *Psychiatrist*: Now, OK, in other words he was sent here for second-degree murder.

(22) *Social Worker*: Oh, well let me go back over it one more time. OK, now the first commitment was in Virginia State Hospital.

(23) *Psychiatrist*: West Virginia.

(24) *Social Worker*: OK. OK. For shooting.

(25) *Psychiatrist*: All right.

In the preceding excerpt the social worker is reminded that presenting oneself expertly is contingent on satisfying the demand of the psychiatrist. In the next excerpt, another social worker is reminded that, for one's theorizing to pass as acceptable, it must ordinarily be agreed to by the psychiatrist. When the psychiatrist suggests that he didn't even pick up on the supposed cue that the social worker is theorizing about, the social worker's line of expert interpretation is laid open to question (line 296). This observed cue is reformulated as a question for the psychiatrist to make sense out of ("Is that a drug reaction?"). Only then is this "slightly off the mark" statement given some status as an expert observation (line 299). The "questionableness" of theoretical inferences by other members is clearly displayed. Others' observations are better formulated in a tentative manner (line 303). All of this stands in stark contrast, however, to the psychiatrist's unchallenged and untentative declaration of clinical facts (line 304).

Excerpt 9-25. From Patient Review 362, Team L

(295) *Social Worker*: Did you notice the . . . [demonstrates visually and audibly the patient's heavy breathing] ?

(296) *Psychiatrist*: No, I didn't

(297) *Psychologist*: What's that?

(298) *Social Worker*: Every time . . . would talk to him his breathing pattern would change and he would go [demonstrates haavy breathing pattern]. He'd get really bad beats, and then when I would start talking to him he'd change and then when you would start talking to him they would get different again. Is that a drug reaction, [name], the rolling of the fingers and uh. . . ?

(299) *Psychiatrist*: No, I think he was a little bit under pressure here. I thought for a minute he was going to, uh, bust out. . . .

(300)  *Psychologist*: I thought he might.

(301)  *Social Worker*: The way he sat there, and he got like this in a very closed . . . position.

(302)  *Psychiatrist*: When I confronted him with the hospitalizations that he had denied, he was silent for a long time.

(303)  *Psychologist*: There is a memory problem, I think.

(304)  *Psychiatrist*: Yes, there's no question that this man is, uh, psychotic, and the psychosis is a manic-depressive and he admits to it and all the symptoms are there, and the manic as paranoid has flavoring . . . OK?

Members are rewarded by being treated as professional coworkers when they show deference to the psychiatrist. Deference is shown through such things as tentatively phrasing theories, elaborating upon psychiatrists' theories, and offering psychiatrists questions by which they can display their high status. When members are not quick to show deference, psychiatrists are quick to withhold expert status. They display one or another of the techniques discussed in this section to put other members in their place. Sometimes this punishment is mild. It may be displayed by the absence of attention to members' theorizing. Often it is subtle. It may be pointed out that a member has misused a technical psychiatric phrase. Occasionally it is less subtle. A member's theorizing may be flatly denied. The impatient tone in a psychiatrist's voice indexes the "fact" that the other is clearly not theorizing like an expert. The topic is abruptly switched away from that being pursued by the "out of line" member. The other is clearly given a warning that if one still wants to salvage any part of an expert identity, he or she had better relinquish theoretical challenges and return to a place of deference.

When considered collectively, the above strategies of status attainment give the psychiatrist a considerable edge over other members. The psychiatrist who successfully uses these strategies comes off as a high status expert who has the ability to mediate the status of others. The one psychiatrist who did not come off with higher status did not successfully employ the final status attainment strategy. He provided no real rewards for others. According to members (in the interviews) and observers (in their notes), this individual entered the review process as a very dominant exponent of a clear medical model. He was also inexperienced in working with interdisciplinary teams. Rather than displaying a control of others' behaviors he did most of the work himself. While this earned him the respect of others as a "hard worker," it did not secure his position as one with highest expert status. Perhaps he was unaware that high status was not taken for granted. This was not the case for the team's psychologist. This individual practiced displays of credentials, clinical skills, and gestures of being in charge and being the team's representative to external agents. Moreover, the psychologist joined in coalition with the social worker to provide a flow of rewards between each other, confirm each other in respective displays of expert identities and deny the psychiatrist the opportunity to guide decisions by withholding status from those who did not fall into his line of theorizing. As such, this was the only team in which a psychiatrist was observed as frequently formulating tentative theories and offering reconciliatory phrasings for other members' acceptance.

If one views the unsuccessful psychiatrist at one end of a continuum and the successful status attainers at the other, one is initially tempted to place the members of the two more "equalitarian" teams somewhere in between. In one sense, this would be an accurate placement. Other members on these teams, by virtue of a more even division of labor, regularly engaged in such high practices as displaying credentials and giving demonstrations of their clinical skills. Furthermore, they were rarely, if ever, interrupted when talking with patients or reviewing records.

In another sense it would be inaccurate or distortive to place the "equalitarian" psychiatrists between unsuccessful and successful "highest status" attainers. Both "equalitarian" psychiatrists were observed to exact subtle but effective control over the direction of final theorizing. When other members offered tentative theories they looked in the direction of the equalitarian psychiatrist. Apparently, approval (or the absense of disapproval) was an important condition for elaborating upon lines of psychiatric reasonings. Moreover, whenever a psychiatrist made a suggestion or offered his own bit of theorizing, these were routinely incorporated into the final diagnostic product. These psychiatrists did not speak as often as the psychiatrists who dominated the whole range of a team's activities. When they did speak, however, they appeared to set the tone and guided the substance of final decisions.

Why equalitarian psychiatrists managed themselves the way they did cannot be readily answered from the available data. Maybe both were simply equalitarian individuals. Clearly both had considerable past experience with team diagnostic sessions. In any event, both generally "got their way" without having to spend many resources. Dominating psychiatrists, on the other hand, were successful in attaining more displays of deference from others. Yet they were also confronted with the problem of having to spend interactional resources defending against the resistance of others. Let us explain.

The attainment of recognizably higher status by psychiatrists put them in positions of higher power. They could and did exercise their will in pushing certain lines of theorizing, even against the resistance of others. The fact that others depended upon them for the granting of expert status provided them with this power. In this sense we see power and dependency as complementary processes. In order to partake in expert status, other members had to exhibit their dependence on psychiatrists through various displays of deference. This did accomplish some sense of expert identity for other members. Yet for persons who, in their own spheres of everyday life, were used to achieving expertness without paying the price of dependency, this practice may have been a problem. This would seemingly have been more the case for most psychologists than for social workers. Psychologists, like psychiatrists, are quite regularly the final arbiters of psychiatric reality. This would be less likely for social workers. Much of their psychiatric work (intake interviews, etc.) is preparatory to others' decision-making. To partake, even as less than equal experts, in a decision-making process, often reserved for psychiatrists (making direct recommendations to court), could possibly elevate their status without increasing ordinary costs.[4]

Given our discussion above, it is not surprising to see psychologists initiate various attempts to balance power and decrease dependency upon psychiatrists. When this occurs, two conditions are generally present. First, the psychologist develops a commitment to a line of theorizing which contradicts that held by a psychiatrist. Second, the psychologist is dependent upon displaying agreement with the psychiatrist in order to be confirmed in an expert identity. The psychologist is placed in the uncomfortable bind of having to publicly display dependency in order to obtain a reward (for example, the accomplishment of an expert identity) which, under other conditions, would be hers or his without such costs. When the discomfirture of such dependency is experienced, the psychologist may attempt to shift the costly imbalance between power and dependency. This appears to be exactly what occurs. Psychologists try out various strategies to decrease the power of the psychiatrists by decreasing their dependency.

In discussing attempts by dependent members to achieve greater power we shall employ a model of power and dependency developed by Richard Emerson.[5] Although this model was the language of "exchange theory," we concur with Prus, who describes the phenomenological utility of Emerson's framework.[6] According to Emerson, dependent actors generally have four options in addressing an imbalance in power and dependency. Two of these involve the object or course of action to which they are committed. Dependent persons can either decide to withdraw their commitment (because it is too costly or not worth it, anyway) or they can try to offer the more powerful person greater rewards if that party will increase (or even show some) commitment to the option to which the dependent party is already committed. Dependent psychologists were observed doing both.

Occasionally psychologists simply appeared to resist interpretations offered by psychiatrists. They withdrew their commitment to contradictory lines of theorizing. This option spared overt displays of dependency on the psychiatrist's line of thinking (that is, showing how he was right and they were wrong). But wouldn't this implicit backing down also jeopardize one's own personal sense of being an expert? By formulating the proposition that "there was nothing one could do anyway," psychologists spared themselves this dilemma.

Some stated that, because of biased cultural expectations, psychiatrists were going to come out on top, anyway. This theme is formulated by a psychologist in the following excerpt.

Excerpt 9-26. From Review Team Questionnaire

Everybody knew it from the beginning that the psychiatrist would be the built-in leader, regardless of what you say about this peer type of thing. I think that that was just sort of a token. I don't think in reality you'd have to plan for it in a different way, in different procedures.

They [psychiatrists] took the authoritarian role, and I'm not saying this in a derogatory way. This is just one of the roles in our culture that an M.D. is not questioned, he's not challenged, and I think it goes along with our cultural role that an M.D. is not challenged . . . even in some things in which he does not have the expertise. He's still looked upon in these areas as though he does have the expertise, and sometimes they respond as though they do have the expertise. Again, this is not personal, I was very fortunate to work with a very well qualified individual. I was very happy with the situation. I thought he did contribute. In fact, he's an excellent man, leading, and a superb performance. But you can't get away from it. That they're not, in our society, that the doctors are not scientists. And people equate them with this. And this is God. I think it's an injustice to the doctors and to us. They are not scientist . . . some, maybe . . . and sometimes we lose fact of this.

You notice some of the expressions when this was announced. That this would be sort of an equal team. It's equal. Only an M.D. is more equal. The psychiatrist is more equal.

At other times, psychologists were able to retain their lines of theorizing but only by offering psychiatrists the status-rewarding option of claiming these theories as if they had thought of them themselves. They would couch their theorizing in the language of disclaimers. They would, in other words, introduce their remarks with lead-ins such as: "Well, I'm not really sure of this, but"; "Tell me, Doctor, do you think its possible that"; "Gee, this is just a hunch, but could it be that. . . ." By offering tentative theorizing in this fashion, members were often successful in increasing psychiatrists' commitments to their lines of theorizing. Yet the option to accept or reject such offerings remained the psychiatrist's. In the long run, this option probably reinforced the imbalance in power and dependency and promoted the likelihood that psychologists would seek other avenues to rectify this uncomfortable experience.

The first two balancing strategies focused on members' commitments to particular avenues of theorizing. The final two are concerned with alternative avenues of reward. The first suggests that the more dependent members could attempt to increase their own alternatives by seeking confirmation for their expert identities outside the existing power set. This is not too practical an alternative. Members were quite literally locked into a limited arena of social interaction. Moreover, as mentioned previously, other actors who do occasionally appear on the scene (for example, hospital staff) tend to display immediate deference to the psychiatrist. The one way that dependent members sometimes employed this strategy was to cite clinical literature or other known expert opinions as the basis for their theorizing. In such cases, they were able both to push their own theorizing and to defend their claims to expertise.

The second alternative reward strategy is for dependent members to join together to limit the powerful parties' own access to high status. Psychiatrists' own situated identities as experts were, after all, also dependent on coming off professionally in the eyes of others. Occasionally psychologists tried to get social workers to "hear" their theorizing as more appropriate than that of the psychiatrist. This attempt at forming a coalition of dependent parties was an important strategy for reducing dependency. When this happened, psychiatrists were likely to respond with reconciliatory, stalemated, or at least "less challenging" reformulations. Note the attempts to form a coalition against a psychiatrist in the following excerpt.

Excerpt 9-27. From Patient Review 71, Team J

(The psychiatrist is challenging the basis for a psychologist's particular theorizing. The psychologist responds by trying to draw the social worker into agreement with his perspective.)

(434)  *Psychiatrist*: Personality disorder worries me the most. Here's a guy who's obviously got a little better than average intelligence, good physical appearance, uh, pretty well put together . . . [continues to document his point for some time and then concludes by stating,] So I think that he's really, uh, probably from the standpoint diagnostically you have to say there's inferential evidence. But you certainly don't have clear-cut evidence. It has to be historical, you know. Interviewing the case he looks like, well, the things he says. . . .

(435)  *Psychologist*: No, I thought it came across in his nonverbal behavior, in his imitations and expressions. What do you think, [name of social worker]? You haven't said anything about that yet, about his affect or nonverbal behavior?

In the preceding discussion, we have observed that psychiatrists, by virtue of their successful employment of certain status evaluation practices, are generally in more powerful positions than other team members. We have also noted certain dependency reduction strategies used (generally by psychologists) to delineate the power of high status psychiatrists. Yet the important issue in considering status and power is not who has more of which per se. Rather we are concerned about the impact of status and power negotiations on the substance of particular psychiatric decisions. In many cases a psychiatrist successfully displays higher status and utilizes this as a resource to push a certain diagnostic theme. When this occurs, the theme is likely to be incorporated into a team's final recommendation. This is partly because other members depend on the psychiatrist to provide them with expert status. They may not challenge his theorizing for that reason alone.

In other cases teams may successfully employ strategies which curtail or at least temporarily readjust the balance of power. We have observed that, at various times, psychologists withdraw or disclaim their own theorizing, and at other times cite outside experts or attempt to form coalitions to defend their theorizing. Depending on each of these strategies, and on how psychiatrists respond, certain lines of theorizing may be dropped, reconciled, stalemated, or modified. In any event, the substance of a psychiatric decision becomes shaped by forces extrinsic to the decision itself. In other words, a patient's diagnostic fate is clearly contingent on the manner in which psychiatric professionals negotiate and defend images of competence and situated identitied as high status experts.

## Anticipating Consequences of Decisions

The way members anticipate the consequences of their action is another major determinant of the substance of a final decision. The key element in this process is the manner in which members arrive at an "awareness" of how others will hear and react to what they have to say. Although this process is most clearly displayed in postinterview discussions, we have already cited numerous examples of it in earlier sections of this report. Let us summarize what has been observed previously and then illustrate the role of anticipating consequences in finalizing theories about patients.

In dealing with anticipating consequences, members appear to present two faces. One is that of public disinterest. The other is that of private concern. The first is an aspect of members' "front stage" management of their expert identities.[7] Teams constantly remind themselves that theirs was an expert, clinical, or behavioral science mission of "discovery" (see excerpt 6-4). They were not to be bogged down by the mundane constraints of judicial decision-making. It was the court, after all, which was really deciding on a patient's fate. They were only "discovering" what a patient was "really" like. This separation between a team's discoveries and the court's adjudications is central to members' "front stage" presentations of themselves. It is typified by the statement of the psychiatrist who suggested: "We can be redundant, say what we mean. If they don't listen, it's not our fault."

Despite a public face of professional disinterest, teams show considerable private or "backstage" concern with how they will be heard. Shortly after the above psychiatrist states, "If they don't listen, it's not our fault," the members of his team begin to discuss whether they should actually call the patient in question a sociopath, for fear that this would mean that he would be retained in maximum security. This is a common occurrence. Teams often express concern about stating a diagnosis "as they really see it" because this may impede a patient's placement in the most appropriate clinical environment. Thus we have observed that members may agree to call a patient "psychopath" even though they believe this to be an inappropriate diagnosis. The problem with this practice is two-fold. First, it places an "untrue" label on a particular patient, a label which then becomes an official part of his diagnostic record. Second, the practice is highly unstandardized. Not all teams used "untrue" labels to get what they wanted. Some simply avoided using problematic labels altogether. One team may include a certain diagnostic term and another may not. Yet, in reading final reports, there is no way of discerning whether this term was actually believed to be clinically relevant. In other words, there is no way to discern what a team "really" had in mind.

Concern about being wrong is another aspect of anticipating consequences which affects the substance of final decisions. We have already observed how this concern guides members in formulating conversative or cautious wordings in their final reports (see excerpt 6-4). In the following excerpt, this concern is translated into practical theorizing. The team is discussing the case of middle-aged black male serving time for armed robbery. Although it is believed that "there is a certain sociopathic element in addition to his paranoid thinking," it is felt that "he has recovered from an acute mental illness" and could be returned to a less restrictive environment. Yet there is some concern that "certain residuals in his basically paranoid personality" may cause him to act out again. If he did, the decision to transfer him away from maximum security would be construed as a costly error by team members. This problem is resolved only when members finally realize that they are not talking about someone who will go back to trial, but about someone who has already been sentenced (line 627). This removes their concern over the costly error of being wrong. The prisoner-patient will not "really" be released, but merely transferred to another restricted setting where, if he gets sick again, he can easily be sent back to maximum security (line 631).

Excerpt 9-28. From Patient Review 163, Team H

(627)   *Psychiatrist*: He is shrewd. There is a certain sociopath element to his paranoid thinking. Uh, I would say that he recovered from an acute mental illness, so there's still some residuals in his basically paranoid personality. I feel that he can stand trial. He was actually sentenced already.

(628)   *Psychologist*: Yeah.

(629)   *Psychiatrist*: So he can be sent back to the correctional institution.

(630)   *Psychologist*: Mmm. Oh, so he would still be confined? Oh, I think that would seem appropriate for him.

(631)   *Psychiatrist*: And if we made an error and he gets sick again he will be in Lima again, right?

(632)   *Psychologist*: Mmm. Mmm. He's got, uh, forty years left in his sentence.

It is important to note that members rarely express concern about concluding that a patient is mentally ill, psychopathic, or dangerous when they "discover" this "fact" in the course of an interview. Perhaps this is because, in part, they have used the past record to formulate their present theorizing. Where they do express a concern over error is in cases which their interviewing leaves them with an impression that the patient is "relatively well," but the record underscores the severity of past problems.

Excerpt 9-29. From Patient Review 210, Team A

(411) *Psychiatrist*: Well, he was pretty well put together in the interview. He seemed in contact with reality, but I feel leery of saying that he's not mentally ill.

(412) *Psychologist*: Because of the record and his present behavior being so inconsistent.

The team excerpted above resolved its dilemma in a typical manner. It included a cautious twist to its final recommendation. It was hence stated that "on the basis of the evaluation of the record and the clinical examination of this patient, it is our opinion that, although he shows, at present, no gross, bizarre psychotic symptoms, his hypertensive, irritable, and cautiously guarded manner are consistent with material in the record showing his psychosis and . . . potential combativeness."

A final aspect of anticipating the reactions of others relates to members' concern that they be heard as expert professionals. This concern translated itself into the formulation of practical rules like that which suggested that "we should never show confusion, even if we are confused" (see excerpt 6-3). This concern, like the anticipation of consequences for patients and the fear of making costly errors, contributes to the shape of final psychiatric decisions. Together these anticipations operate as central features of the context in which decisions are made. They are worked with and used to form the substance of a diagnostic recommendation. Yet, like the influence of status and power, their impact is reflectively lost in the aftermath of a decision. Once again, the work that goes into formulating decisions is disguised by "objective" appearance of the final product.

## Individuation of Troubles: Discounting Cultural, Class, and Political Reality

The successful "discovery" of psychiatric reality requires that members sort through a large amount of written, verbal, and nonverbal stimuli and isolate the individual roots of a patient's problems. This theorizing about individual problems routinely discredits the validity of social accounts for patients' present situations. Specifically it requires clinicians to discount explanations that may have little to do with "psychiatric," but a lot to do with cultural, class, or political reality.

Attempts at the individuation of troubles present a problem for psychiatric team members and patients alike. Often this means that patients' own accounts of their problems must be denigrated. For instance, a patient may come from a cultural setting in which much of the world is interpreted through notions of "fate" or "chance." A patient may have lived in a class setting in which violence is construed as a "normal" response to personal affronts and challenges. A patient may presently live in a setting where his or her "disruptive" or "deviant" behaviors are provoked by the discriminatory or abusive actions of those "in charge." Actually, most Lima State patients come from, have lived in, and presently dwell in all three such settings. Nonetheless, accounts concerning their behaviors using fatalistic cultural notions, class-based definitions of violence, or a political analysis of hospital pressures are routinely interpreted as evidence of delusional thinking, denials of responsibility, and paranoid reactions. Thus, attempts to fit patients into theories about psychiatric reality systematically discredit the other realities by which patients live.

My suggestion that psychiatric theorizing denigrates social accounts does not imply that members never consider cultural, class, or political variables. At various points, members were observed making statements such as the following: "Well, we can't be shocked. We have to consider that this [incest] is more common among these [mountain] people. It doesn't have the same moral meaning." "Boy, I'll tell you. He comes from a part of Cleveland, mmm [where] I'd carry a gun around." "You know, the first-degree murder thing, it was because he killed a white man. If it was a black it would have been different."

At first glance, like those above, the statements appear to widen the understanding of a patient's troubles, opening the door to other social accounts for her or his "deviance." This is not, however, how such statements are used in practical psychiatric theorizing. These statements can accomplish a sympathetic viewing of a patient, but are not allowed to pass as theoretical accounts of her or his troubles. They may help a team "see" that patient as a cooperative, unfortunate, or honest person. They will not help explain what her or his "real" problems are and why she or he did what was done. This is evidenced in the discussion excerpted below.

The following case involves a young black male who was paralyzed from the waist down from a shooting incident several years past. He is presently charged with carrying a concealed weapon. His parents, who believed he was acting "too wild" and disturbed around the house, reported him to the police. Their testimony in court was apparently a key element in his commitment to Lima State Hospital until restored to reason. During the interview, the patient was composed but stated that he would probably continue to carry a weapon in order to protect his property and that he had refused to take his medication because it made him sick.

After the patient left the room, the psychologist discussed signs of paranoid schizophrenia and expressed concern over the patient's intent to carry a gun, his almost "unnatural fear" of someone's taking his property, and his "perceived enmity or hostility towards his family." The psychiatrist elaborated upon this, stating: "This is abnormal. You don't carry a knife around to stab someone because you feel you'll get stabbed. This man was disturbed." The social worker initially seemed less sure of this line of theorizing. Shouldn't the case be seen in relation to a sociocultural milleu in which gun-carrying would be seen as "normal" (line 558)? The psychiatrist agreed, but then efficiently managed the conversation so that it was recognized that these broader issues were really not the patient's problem. His problem was psychiatrically refocused at the individual level. His disturbed behavior at home was the "real" issue (line 567). The social worker "sees" this and returns to theorizing about the patient's individualized trouble. Late in the interview, the social worker theorizes entirely at the level of psychiatric reality. The patient's disturbed behavior is talked about as a form of compensation for his physical disability. Social accountings are discarded in favor of individualized psychiatric explanations.

Excerpt 9-30. From Patient Review 212, Team G

(556)    *Social Worker*: Uh, I agree that carrying, I think we ought to know that another thing too. This is a relatively young black. I think he's got an attitude that is I think indicative to many blacks today. Which—he looks at other, maybe a white person here comes and says, "Well, look, you know, why are you carrying a gun?" I mean the, I'm not saying he's looking at it from this perspective, you know, but, "Look, why shouldn't I carry a gun? I mean, whites carry guns. Look what you did in Vietnam." Now, I could be off base on this, but in. . . . You have to look from whence he came. Like, I know Detroit. It would not be abnormal to carry, to walk around with, a gun.

(557)    *Psychiatrist*: OK. Now I'm not disagreeing.

(558)    *Social Worker*: Because you don't know what's going to happen. I mean, that fear in Detroit is so great, and the grabbing-of-power movement is so great, that people do carry weapons.

(559)    *Psychiatrist*: Well, fine. What I was saying: this, all what you said is, I, I take it one hundred percent.

(560)    *Social Worker*: Mmm.

(561)    *Psychiatrist*: I take it into extreme whatever you're saying.

(562)    *Social Worker*: Mmm.

(563)    *Psychiatrist*: But I bring it home and I come to your immediate parents.

(564)    *Social Worker*: And I agree with you there.

(565)    *Psychiatrist*: All right.

(566)    *Social Worker*: Fine, because that's where. . . .

(567)  *Psychiatrist*: And they felt the need that their son is not an adult, not controlled.

(568)  *Social Worker*: I agree with you.

(569)  *Psychiatrist*: And he's off.

(570)  *Social Worker*: I agree with you.

(571)  *Psychiatrist*: And this is the time where they called. . . .

(572)  *Social Worker*: Yeah, they called.

(573)  *Psychiatrist*: That's right. They called for help from the [police].

(574)  *Social Worker*: Mmm.

(At this point the psychologist enters the conversation and engages the psychiatrist in a series of lengthy exchanges about the nature of the patient's family situation and the patient's legal status. When the psychiatrist calls for a final formulation of the team's recommendations, the social worker offers the following "individualized theorizing.")

(680)  *Social Worker*: I was just saying how that his rebelliousness might be a form of compensating for. . . .

(681)  *Psychiatrist*: Oh, yes. Oh, well, yes. Yes, of course it is. All this. . . .

(682)  *Social Worker*: Carrying a gun may give him part of his manhood.


The preceding excerpt represents an instance in which social accounts are introduced but then subsequently neutralized in favor of psychiatric reasoning. In most cases, a patient's attempt to account for her or his troubles in social terms is rejected from the onset. Often this rejection seems sociologically naive. In one case a team asked a lower-class male patient what he would do if he were on a public bus and someone came up and started calling him obscene names. The patient stated that it depended on whether the person was a male or female. If it was a male, he said that the person deserved to get punched. Such an answer seems somewhat "typical" from the perspective of a culture and class, wherein the possibility of violence and rigid distinctions between expectations for males and females are taken as commonplace. From the vantage point of psychiatric diagnosticians, however, the situation looked quite different. Team members noted the distinction between males and females "as if" it were evidence of the patient's ambivalence toward women and saw the fact that the event might precipitate violence as indicative that "his judgment remains impulsive."

In the case described above the team denigrates the value of a patient's cultural and class-based accounting. What the patient saw as a "normal" response to a troublesome situation, team members saw as "pathological." This applies to descriptions of political reality as well. When patients presented themselves as political victims of exploitive hospital practices, their stories were typically discredited. In one case, a patient stated that the reason he had been discharged was because staff accused him of forwarding a petition which "undermined hospital policy." The team searching for the individual roots for his problem concluded that this was "indicative of some kind of marginal adjustment, barely adjusted or something, because he gives a good excuse for everything." In another case, a patient's story about being victimized by a "crackpot psychiatrist," by staff discrimination and the lack of treatment in Lima State Hospital and at a home for delinquents, which he characterized as more of a jail than a school, were all taken as documents of his need to rationalize and drive to manipulate. In response to a story about sexual abuse at the hospital by a woman (who, in fact, had testified at previous public hearings on this matter), a team showed interest but was reluctant to accept this as the reason for the patient's "real" problems within the institution. Her statements were taken as evidence of delusions and projections of her own homosexual identity to others. As the team suggested in formulating its final opinion, "Some of this goes on but mostly it's just her delusions."

The preceding examples were presented as illustrations of a prevailing pattern. Potentially plausible cultural, class, and political accounts are struck down in favor of a focus on the individual roots of deviance. This is an important element in the formulation of final diagnostic decisions. Yet, as with the negotiation of status and power and the anticipation of the consequences of making certain recommendations, this factor remains behind the scenes. It is always present as a contextual or indexical constraint regarding what members will allow to pass as valid theorizing, yet it is never stated in so many words. It remains as an implicit guide to the construction of psychiatric reality.

### Transforming Theorizing into "Expert" Findings

Once members agreed on what it was that they "discovered" they set forth their findings in a summary report to the court. This was the final step in the review process. This final step, however, entailed more than a simple rehashing of what went on in the review and what members believed they learned about a patient. It is rather a transformation of what members did and concluded into a highly specialized professional language which presents itself as an "objective" and "expert" description of a patient's individual psychiatric reality. Gone are all traces of the interactional process by which members formulated "senses," "hunches," and "theories" about patients. Remaining is an impressive array of terminology which describes the patient in terms of "syndromes" and "symptoms."

Much of this chapter has concerned itself with the process through which members take empirical inferences and convert them into theoretical statements. In final reports, the exact nature of members' empirical inferences are left out.

Their theoretical statements are honed up into tightly worded, expertly defined opinions and recommendations. Gone are those "empirical" inferences such as members' reliance on the "long look" of aggressive homosexuality, a requested joke which revealed a patient's inner turmoil, or a patient's "rationalizing" story about how she had been sexually abused and mistreated. Nor was it reported that such items as the "clearly" agitated glance, the "welling-up eyes," the "obvious" attempt to use one's good looks, or the "manipulative" desire for school, all constituted the evidence by which members retrospectively justified their decisions to each other. Nor was the influence of status and power, the anticipation of certain consequences or the discounting of class, cultural, and political reality, ever cited as shaping decisions. All of these interactional elements were left aside. In their place, members substituted the technical language of psychiatric diagnosis.

The legal audience which received the expert opinions of psychiatric team members missed much by only receiving opinions worded in objective diagnostic nomenclature. This nomenclature was more than a professional shorthand. It was also a disguise for the subjective inferences and social interactions which produced it. For instance, in reading the final report on a particular patient, one learns that the patient shows "a definite schizoid type personality, with anti-social personality traits and the fact that the defendant has always expressed his views openly with defiance, and with the idea of having an open mind, demanding and needing freedom, and feeling that laws are to be broken." What one does not learn is that it was this patient's complaints about "unjust" regulations at a boys' reformatory and his insistence that everybody has broken a law at some time which led members to formulate their recommendations accordingly (see excerpt 8-26).

Throughout the text of this chapter we have cited numerous cases in which retrospective and reconciliatory inferences and modifications in theorizing, due to a variety of social contingencies, are left out of the explicit frame of a final psychiatric decision. All of these things go into the framing of a particular decision, but are in the final product, hidden by the frame itself. This is the essential thing to remember about this last step in the patient review process. It is a step which transforms loose indexical theorizing into tight, reflexively realized "fact." The interactionally determined basis for a conclusion is lost in the reading of the expertly stated conclusion itself. Ad hoc theories become objective findings. The many steps which generate a decision are disguised by the one step which announces that decision.

## Notes

1. Members' rules for handling the dilemma of contradictory information are differently related to the "denying" and "admitting" modes. These rules are

essentially irrelevant to patients in the "displaying" mode. After all, displays of illness only provide grounds for elaborating upon the problems that members have already theorized about.

2. In interactional terms, we are suggesting that since powerful parties are able to get their way even against the resistance of others, they need not anticipate the reaction of others or "take the role of others" and adjust accordingly. According to Franks: " 'Structurally legitimated' power can function in place of role taking to overcome the resistance of others." Cf. David D. Franks, "Social Power, Role Taking, and the Structure of Imperceptiveness: Toward a Redefinition of False Consciousness," *Annals of Phenomenological Sociology* 1 (1976): 107.

3. This matter of thematizing purposes-at-hand has already been given considerable attention in Chapter 6. Members' primary purposes-at-hand were described as both trying to make (psychiatric) sense out of patients and trying to appear (expertly) sensible before each other.

4. In this sense psychiatrists not only display the power of reward and punishment, but also what Raven calls "referent power." Cf. B.H. Raven, "Social Influence and Power," in I.D. Steiner and M. Fishbein, eds., *Current Studies in Social Psychology* (New York: Holt, Rinehart, and Winston, 1965).

5. The complementary positioning of power and dependency is underscored by Emerson. Power is conceived of in terms of having less motivational investment or commitment to a particular course of action and more interactional alternatives for achieving a particular end than one's dependent role partner. Cf. Richard Emerson, "Power and Dependence Relations," *American Sociological Review* 27 (February 1962): 31-41.

6. Robert C. Prus, "Resisting Designations: An Extension of Attribution Theory into a Negotiated Contact," *Sociological Inquiry* 45(1):10.

7. This is an excellent example of how members "take the role" of imagined others through a process of negotiated conversation about how others will respond.

**Part IV
Summary**

# 10 Concluding the Study: Implications of Viewing Psychiatric Diagnosis as a Practical Accomplishment

*The growing army of social workers, psychologists, psychiatrists . . . etc., constitutes a stratum with a precise interest in ensuring a flow of persons defined as deviant. The training undergone by such specialists creates a stratum whose aim it is to discover "out there" in the empirical world those sorts of people they have been trained to see.*

> John Lofland, *Deviance and Identity* (Englewood Cliffs, N.J.: 1969), p. 136.

In this study I have sought to display and analyze the production of expert psychiatric knowledge by agents of social control. Unlike most previous studies the work here has not directly concerned itself with whether predictive psychiatric decisions are reliable or valid. The past literature already suggests that they are not. Our concern has been with the process of interaction between official agents of social control and potential targets of deviant labeling. In this final chapter, I shall briefly summarize our major findings, outline theoretical implications for the study of deviance, and discuss pragmatic implications for the formulation of mental health policy.

## What the Study Concludes

The most significant finding of our study is that *diagnostic decisions are inherently bound to and thus dependent upon a variety of ongoing social or social psychological processes that may have little to do with the psychiatric troubles or emotional disturbances of patients.* The operation and impact of these inherent social processes have been observed in each of the three major stages of psychiatric decision-making. Thus, we have noted that:

1. *In previewing patients, diagnosers typically employed a logic of discovery that is best described by the term "theorizing."* Review team members did not ordinarily make simple notations of "fact." They began immediately to formulate stories about patients' present psychiatric status by making theoretical inferences from official descriptions of past confinements.

217

2. *In interviewing patients, diagnosers approached patients with a particular cognitive style at variance with that associated with display of talk in everyday life.* In diagnostic conversations patients' verbal accounts were not allowed to pass as taken for granted, as prestructured, or as intersubjective. They were theoretically scrutinized for documentation that patients live in a non-everyday reality characterized by psychiatric disturbances.

3. *In postviewing patients, diagnosers employ a "logic of justification" (to display the documentary grounds for decisions already made) and a "logic of reconciliation" (to display consensus and continuity in response to the resistance of others).* Members did not systematically weigh or assess supportive and contradictory pieces of evidence. They formulated and reformulated decisions by searching for evidence which buttressed what was already "known" about a particular patient.

These general conclusions regarding the diagnostic process may be broken down into more specific observations of the interactional work involved in producing a particular psychiatric decision. These have been spelled out in considerable detail in Chapters 5 through 9. We shall not attempt to replicate such detail in this final chapter. These observations can, however, be formulated in terms of a series of empirical generalizations. The first set of these generalizations encompasses what we shall call "the essential features" of members' interactions with each other and with patients. These are necessary elements, without which diagnostic decision-making would not be what it is—a social construction of a psychiatric reality. The production of a particular diagnosis is dependent, in part, upon each of four such essential features of members' interaction. These include:

1. *the manner in which diagnosers formulate theoretical inferences from the past record* (Chapter 7);
2. *the manner in which diagnosers manage "theoretically styled" psychiatric interview talk through such practices as selective questioning, selective hearing, selective offering of accounts, and the pushing of idiosyncratic themes* (Chapter 8);
3. *the manner in which diagnosers use justificatory and reconciliatory logic in finalizing psychiatric theorizing about patients* (Chapter 9);
4. *the manner in which diagnosers use the abstract and technical terminology of a specialized psychiatric language to transform negotiated decisions into "objective" sounding expert findings* (Chapter 9).

The features of members' interactions outlined above depict social processes that are the essence of what goes on in the production of psychiatric diagnoses. Yet, each of these essential features are vague or indeterminate. Their specificity depends on the manner in which each is shaped or formed by what we shall refer to as "contingent features" of members' interactions. In other words, the concrete (observable and observed) enactment of each essential feature is dependent, in part, upon the outcomes of a number of other contingent social processes. These include:

1. *the manner in which diagnosers formulate assumptions about what it is that they are legally mandated to do* (Chapters 6 and 7);
2. *the manner in which diagnosers formulate assumptions about the meaning of relevant clinical categories* (Chapters 6 and 7);
3. *the manner in which diagnosers employ different professional and personal perspectives on psychiatric diagnosis and its consequences* (Chapter 5);
4. *the manner in which diagnosers perceive different styles of a patient's diagnostic presentation of his or herself* (Chapter 8);
5. *the manner in which diagnosers negotiate different displays of expert professional status and the use of power* (Chapter 9);
6. *the manner in which diagnosers anticipate different consequences of announcing certain diagnostic decisions* (Chapter 9);
7. *the manner in which members construct different individuated theories of a patient's psychiatric troubles* (Chapter 9).

The list of contingent interactional features is more specific or closer to what members concretely do than is the list of essential features. Nonetheless, each contingent feature also contains a certain vagueness or indeterminacy. Each is stated in terms of "the manner in which" members perform this or that social act (formulate, employ, perceive, negotiate, etc.). What, however, determines the specific "manner in which" something actually happens? Are there rules which govern members' specific choices about the "manner in which" contingent features are structured? If so, have we discovered these rules?

My analysis suggested that the contingent features of members' interactions "appear to be" structured, and that the way they are structured influences the way that the essential features are enacted. It additionally suggests that the contingent features "appear to be" structured in terms of members' rules regarding which option to choose in a particular situation. These rules "appear to govern" such things as what to do when one wants to control the consequences of one's decisions, how to perceive a patient who resists one's selective theorizing, or what to make of a patient's use of cultural, class, or political accounts for one's troubles. At various points in the preceding chapters such "rules" have been specifically formulated in terms of propositions stating, "If this, then that." Shouldn't we then complete this summary of findings by listing the rules governing each contingent feature? We would then have reached the conclusion that members' rules give structure to "contingent features" which, in turn, give structure to "essential features" which, in turn, produce diagnostic decisions.

If we were to treat members' rules in the manner suggested above, we would appear to be introducing an explanatory structure resembling Kaplan's model of patterned or "concatenated theorizing."[1] According to this model, a given dependent variable is understood to be codetermined by the simultaneous interaction of a number of independent variables. If we were using this model, it would be suggested that a diagnostic decision, an essential feature, or a contingent feature (depending upon our level of analysis) be considered as a dependent variable. Other features would thus become independent variables, interacting with each other in co-determining the outcome or direction of the dependent variable. In this sense, we would be proposing a model of "triple concatenation." Independent variables at one level of analysis would be treated as dependent variables at another.

A concatenated model might be of some help in "spatially" depicting the interactional processes with which we are concerned. Yet, this *is not* the model being proposed. This model distorts rather than clarifies our findings. In order to employ a concatenated model one must have observed that the features of interaction are, in fact, governed by specific rules. One must have discovered that there are rules which give structure to members' interactions with each other. This *we have not* observed. Rather, we *have observed the opposite*. Members' interactions only *appear to be* rule governed. They *are not*, in actuality, rule governed. The appearance that rules exist and provide structure is itself a worked-at product. Rules are embedded as "ad hoc" displays of rationality or accountability in the occasions of their use. The articulation of rules is an essential element in members' logic of justification. It is through the formulation of rules that "the things that clinicians saw" are converted into "the indicators of a particular type of psychiatric reality."

Psychiatric team members displayed rules concerning how certain things were known about a patient's psychiatric reality. For instance, if a patient was young and had been previously labeled a psychopath, team members were likely to articulate some "rule of evidence" which would justify a diagnosis of psychopathy based upon such criteria. They would make some statement such as, "Yeah, this guy's got age against him. You know, there's no stopping psychopaths until they burn out with age." The articulation of such a rule, however, is "ad hoc" or bound to the context in which it occurred. If, in the same case, a powerful psychiatrist had noted "some insight on this guy's part," the rule of age might be reconciliatorily dropped in favor of a rule suggesting that "because of the existence of some insight it is evident that the patient is not a standard psychopath." Thus, the articulation of rules, like the "discovery" of indicators, is intrinsically bound to and contingent upon everything else that is going on between members at a given time.

The "ad hoc" production of rules was essential in light of members' two primary purposes-at-hand, to make sense of patients and appear expertly sensible. Together these purposes-at-hand imply that there must be something "out there" to which one's discoveries correspond and to which one's expert methodologies lead. By invoking rules for making sense and appearing sensible, members were able to create and sustain the sense (or appearance) that these purposes were accomplished. The articulation or display of rules provided members with the sense that their work was structured in terms of things that are "really there." It enabled psychiatric professionals to produce a sense of structured social reality for both patients and themselves.

The manner in which members provided a sense of structure for their decision-making was inherently indexical. By this we mean that the manner in which some facet of psychiatric reality was discovered as "being there" (dangerousness, mental illness, psychopathy, etc.) was inevitably codetermined by what else members were doing in relation to each other. For this reason we shall not attempt to review the many uses of rules by which members accounted for why they did what they did. Our description and analysis of this process occupies many pages in the preceding chapters.

It would be inefficient to summarize individual displays of rules at this point. More importantly, simply to list the various rules by which members gave a sense of structure to "the manner in which" they formulated this assumption, negotiated that indicator of status, or anticipated such and such a consequence of making a certain recommendation, would be to wrench their interactional work from the context in which it was bound. In our preceding analysis we have tried to preserve as much as this context as possible.

One way in which our analysis has probably distorted the indexical nature of psychiatric decision-making was by dealing with various contingent interactional features one at a time. In actuality, these processes (negotiating status, formulating assumptions, anticipating consequences, etc.) are enacted simultaneously. Thus, the results of certain status arrangements impact upon the formulation of certain assumptions, which impact upon the anticipation of likely consequences. In other words, each feature of the decision-making process partially shapes and is partially shaped by all else that is going on among the psychiatric team members.

While a description and analysis of the indexical nature of psychiatric decision-making is a most important finding, also significant is the documentation of the "unnoticed reflexivity" which guides the process. At each stage of the diagnostic process, the work that produces the "manner in which" psychiatric reality is given the appearance of being structured is lost behind the sense of structure itself. Collective reformulations of theorizing in terms of reconciliation or deference are not remembered. What is remembered is the product of interactional work—the appearance of a "rule-guided" recognition of psychiatric reality is reflexively covered up by the accomplished "objectivity" of what has been discovered. The end not only justifies the means, but also disguises its essential (social) features.

## Theoretical Implications: What the Study Means
## for the Conceptualization of Deviance

*Support for the Social Reaction Perspective*

The results of our study appear to clearly support the social reaction perspective on deviance. Psychiatric decisions were found to be dependent on the manner in which designated diagnostic agents engaged in or negotiated a set of essential and contingent features of social interaction. It was only through such interaction that decisions were actually made and recognized as such by psychiatric professionals. Without such social interactions patients' deviant identities would remain essentially unformulated. This is not to say that a patient's behavior was not used in assessing psychiatric reality. As we observed in Chapter 8 a patient's mode of self-presentation is an important ingredient in constructing psychiatric theorizing. It is not, however, an isolated or primarily important ingredient. It is at all times contextually or indexically related to the other interactional processes that are simultaneously occurring (negotiations of status and power, anticipation of consequences, formulation of assumptions, etc.). As such, the generation of a deviant label is seen as inherently social.

How significant a patient's actual behavior is in producing a diagnostic decision is bound to what team members perceive as most relevant to a particular point in time. Relevancy, in turn, appears dependent on members' success in achieving their two primary purposes-at-hand. If, for instance, a team chose not to read a patient's record before interviewing, what the person actually did in the interview may have been more important than if the team already "knew" the patient from her or his past record. The importance of this may be emphasized by members' need to make clinical sense of a patient. In practice, of course, this was not always the case. Teams not previewing records often displayed a tendency, an ability, to "wait and see" what a patient's behavior meant, until they could retrospectively interpret it in terms of the record. Moreover, against the resistance of a powerful psychiatrist other members would often "selectively hear" only those statements which fit with the psychiatrist's theorizing. Such a hearing may deemphasize other aspects of a patient's behavior, although it may facilitate the realization of members' second purpose-at-hand, "appearing expertly sensible." In any case, we have observed that interpretations of what a patient is "really" like are inherently bound to a social process in which perception of a patient's actual behavior is only one interdependent element.

*The Utility of the Ethnomethodological Approach*

In addition to providing general support for the social reaction perspective, this study has underscored the utility of this perspective's "ethnomethodological" strand. An ethnomethodological focus has allowed us to bypass the so-called "correctness" issue. In Chapter 2 we saw how this issue confused the debate between labeling theory and an "objectivist" perspective on deviance. As distinct from either labeling theory or the objectivist perspective, our ethnomethodological interests have guided us away from choosing sides in the battle over which set of factors (social or medical) better explain the prevalence of deviance. Our research has treated neither social nor medical factors as explanatory factors. Rather, we have been concerned with how clinicians themselves "discover" such factors and produce "rules" which appear to govern their use. Employing this perspective we have seen both social and medical factors produced as accounting or discounting for deviance.

For psychiatric professionals, the relative importance of different factors (social or medical) in accounting for the recognition of norm violations is tied to an ongoing process of sense-making and appearing sensible. Thus, by viewing psychiatric decisions as products of negotiated interaction, I am not suggesting that "things" such as mental illness, dangerousness, or need for maximum security are not "really there." Certainly they are "really there" for members. What we have found, however, is that the way they "become really there" is inherently bound to the interactional practices of members themselves.

The indexical treatment of diagnostic resources is as much the case for "social" as it is for "medical" variables. In Chapter 2 we observed that sociologists associated with the labeling perspective have often denigrated the independent reality of such "medical variables" as hallucinations, psychological testing scores, and official psychiatric records. Yet these same theorists have treated such "social variables" as class, status, organizational context, or professional socialization as if they existed independently of the occasions of their use. In the present study we have discovered no warrant to treat either set of variables as existing independently. Both are used at various times and with varying degrees of importance by members in making sense and appearing sensible. Moreover, the manner in which social and medical factors are used shifts with shifts in the practical relevance of one or another contingent features of members' interaction.

As an illustration of the indexical use of social factors, consider members' use of "social status." Much of Chapter 8 concerned itself with the manner in which status is interactionally achieved. It is not some independent variable which affects members. It is a resource which members use to affect each other. Thus, status is formulated in a different way when members appear to agree on certain assumptions about their legal mandate from when they appear to disagree about the consequences of a particular decision. So also, the meaning of a hallucination, the importance of one's clinical training, the amount of medication, or the interpretation of a "long look of homosexuality," etc., are all dependent on the indexical context in which various interactional features are being displayed and used. In other words, depending on what else is happening the use of a particular social or medical factor may happen in this or that manner. Our previous listing of contingent features of members' interactions is a way of suggesting what else is probably happening at any given point in diagnostic time.

*Expanding the Ethnomethodological Approach*

Besides displaying the utility of an ethnomethodological approach, I have also demonstrated the benefits of expanding this approach to include a systematic consideration of such matters as interests, identities, and resistances. Interests and identities were conceptualized in terms of members' dual purposes-at-hand. Resistance was formulated in terms of whatever anyone else was doing to advance her or his own interests or situate a particular identity at the expense of another.

By expanding the ethnomethodological focus we were able to expand our appreciation of complex social reality. Thus, members were understood not only as constructing realities, but also as negotiating ways of making sense and "coming off" as sensible, even when others act as constraining forces. How all of this happens was, of course, the subject of our previous analysis. In concluding, let us simply observe that the treatment of interests, identities, and resistances offers the promise of enriching ethnomethodology's understanding of what actors do in everyday life.

## Pragmatic Implications: What the Study Means for Mental Health Policy

The finding that psychiatric decision-making is inherently tied to a process of negotiated interaction has significant implications for mental health policy. As we have consistently observed, what goes on between psychiatric professionals in a collective process is often more important in determining the shape of a diagnostic recommendation than is what goes on with a patient. Yet, the particular shape of a decision has the most serious of consequences for patients. With this in mind, I turn to the pragmatic implications of this study. I shall confine this discussion to three areas: an additional comment on the reliability and validity of psychiatric decision-making, the political consequences of the type of diagnostic procedures observed, and some suggestions for something better.

*Reliability and Validity: A Footnote*

This study was in no way designed as a direct assessment of either the reliability or validity of psychiatric diagnosis. In the opening chapter I did, however, suggest that my analysis might provide feedback on clinicians' "criteria-in-use" in formulating decisions about such matters as mental illness, dangerousness, incompetency, need for maximum security, and psychopathy. I also suggested that an examination of these "criteria-in-use" might enhance our understanding of social interaction as an intermediate variable in experimental and/or longitudinal assessments of reliability and validity. The discussion of members' actual "criteria-in-use" (particularly in Chapter 5) has provided information in these areas. It has also provided some "indirect" feedback on the issues of reliability and validity. This feedback is summarized in the following paragraphs.

We have observed numerous inconsistencies in members' criteria-in-use both within and between teams. Within teams it was suggested that criteria are not applied uniformly from patient to patient. For one patient the "fact" that she or he was attractive, young, intelligent, desirous of college, eager to get married, or committed to getting a good job on the "outside" could be taken as positive indicators of relatively few psychiatric troubles. For the next patient these same "facts" may be taken as evidence of manipulative tendencies and the individual may be seen as a dangerous psychopath. Moreover, the reason that these differences in diagnostic interpretations occur may have little to do with a patient's actual behavior, but a lot to do with what I have referred to as the "essential" and "contingent" features of team members' interaction.

Numerous differences among teams in assumptions and diagnostic practices have also been noted. For instance, while all teams were observed to rely on records of past violence in determining dangerousness, it was observed that teams varied considerably in their emphasis on the importance of past violence, as well as in their assessment of the "recency" of violence and the significance of "dangerous delusions." Moreover, most teams also viewed the "lack of control" during interviews as a necessary component of diagnosing violence. Yet, teams varied greatly in what was taken as an indicator of "lack of control." Some teams focused on whether patients showed insight to past acts of violence, while others relied on such diverse criteria as the assessment of dreams and fantasies, the results of psychological testing, or the "observed" repression of anger. Some members even suggested that "personal" definitions, such as whether one would want a particular patient as a neighbor, were the key determinants of judgments about dangerousness.

Teams' "criteria-in-use" also varied in determining the need for maximum security. Although most clinicians viewed this as an outcome of the prediction of dangerousness, some teams placed a premium on such matters as the length of time that a person has been hospitalized and records of previous escapes by those who were "potentially assaultive." Yet teams were, perhaps, most inconsistent in considering the fate of the so-called "psychopathic offender." Teams varied in whether psychopaths were considered treatable. Teams that believed these persons were not treatable still varied in whether they felt incorrigible psychopaths should stay at Lima, depending on their age, the length of their confinement, and whether or not they were becoming "more restrained." Teams also varied in whether they should label nonpsychopaths as psychopaths so that these persons (who can benefit from treatment) will get treatment. They were similarly inconsistent in whom they would label "real" psychopaths, whom they didn't want to stay at the hospital (because they could not benefit from treatment).

My documentation of inconsistencies represents, if only indirectly, the unreliability of psychiatric diagnosis. More importantly, it grounds the basis for this unreliability in the network of social interactions which constitute the very essence of psychiatric decision-making. These observations also suggest a certain footnote on the topic of validity. Do psychiatric diagnosis measure what they say they measure—the psychiatric reality of patients? My analysis suggests that they do not. At least, the degree to which they do measure the "internal mental status" of patients is inherently contingent upon a complex process of social interaction of negotiation over issues that have little or nothing to do with what a patient is "really" like (negotiations over status, or the anticipation of consequences, etc.). Thus, the actual assessment of a patient is not and cannot be separated from what makes diagnosis what it is—a social construction of psychiatric reality.

*Political Consequences: Managing Deviance as "Individual" Pathos*

The psychiatric predictions of dangerousness or the need for confinement in a maximum-security environment are acts which are inherently political. They represent the process by which it is professionally decided to curtail one individual's present freedom for the purpose of guarding another's future safety. In this study, we have examined the interactional practices which both constitute and conceal the intrinsic social structuring of this process. In doing so, it has been discovered that this process is systematically biased in favor of preserving the present balance of power within the criminal justice system and related agencies of social control. Let me explain.

One of the foremost conclusions of this study is that what diagnosticians did and did well was to "produce" individual theories of psychiatric trouble. Clearly, this particular type of diagnostic production has significant political consequences. In constructing these individual theories of deviance, diagnosticians affix the blame for violent, harmful, or dangerous behavior on the psychiatric realities or "individual pathos" of patients. Such practical theorizing was seen to preserve the expert professional identity of psychiatric diagnosticians. Yet in Chapter 9 it was discovered that the individuation of psychiatric troubles also denigrates attempts by patients to "socially account" for psychiatric problems. It requires clinicians to discount explanations that may have little to do with "psychiatric reality" but a lot to do with cultural, class, or political reality.

In the construction of psychiatric diagnoses, potentially plausible cultural, class, and political accounts are struck down in favor of explanations that favor a focus on the individual roots of social deviance. This practice has important implications not only for the diagnostic fate of individual patients, but also for the system of social control as a whole. The present system of criminal justice is, after all, constructed on the principle of "individual pathology." It is the individual offender who is held culpable, and he or she alone, for violations against the sociolegal order of things. The work of diagnostic professionals reinforces the operations of that system. Their work in "discovering" the individual roots of dangerousness and need for maximum security, and their denigration of cultural, class, and political accounts regarding these matters, underscore the assumption of "individual pathology" behind the present handling of crimes and violence. Thus, while manifestly accomplishing a sense of expert identity, diagnosticians simultaneously perpetuate the interests of the larger order of social control.

It appears that the psychiatric assessment of dangerousness and need for maximum security is a political act by which accounts of violence are stripped of their social and political meaning. Actions (past, present, and possibly future) are wrenched from their sociopolitical context. They are interpretively converted by psychiatric diagnosticians into theories of personal pathology. Moreover, the empirical basis for judgments about "individual pathology" are transformed or mystified by the use of an abstract professional language. The management of this language helps to secure an expert identity for its users. It also serves to mask essentially moral or political judgments in the logic and rhetoric of psychiatric expertise. As such, the whole process of making psychiatric predictions about who needs to be confined functions to support a criminal justice system, emphasizing individuals rather than systems, or sociopolitical contexts, as the real perpetrators of violence and harm.

In observing the "political interests" served by the prediction process, it is not suggested that psychiatric diagnosticians consciously victimize anyone, deliberately denigrate others' versions of reality, or intentionally participate in the maintenance of a particular system of social control. It is suggested that these things happen. They appear earnest in viewing their work as that of discovery. They appear capable of simultaneously thematizing ideals of reform and social control, while expressing confidence in their abilities to handle work which is admittedly difficult. It is not their good or bad motives that are at issue, but the consequences of what they do and how they do it. These observations are made so that psychiatric professionals (and by extension all of us) may confront the consequences of the way that professional activity contributes to the process of social control and to the maintenance of the existing political order.

Despite the "good" intentions of the psychiatric professionals, psychiatric predictions of need for confinement have "bad" consequences and should be abandoned. They have not proved themselves better than predictions derived by random chance. They have proved themselves unwarrantedly conservative in producing high rates of false positives and in denigrating the indigenous accounts of others' realities. Worst of all, they have provided reinforcement for an assumption within the criminal justice system which systematically prevents the realization of social justice—the principle of "individual pathology." This principle reifies an individualistic view of the world, while discrediting the conception that humans' potentials, possibilities, and practices are intricately related to the fates of the collectivities in which they live and find both meaning and existence.[2] Through relatively exclusive adherence to this principle, the criminal justice system is able to isolate violence in the acts of individuals. Ignored are political meanings of such acts. These meanings may vary from representing fairly deliberate statements about imbalances in privilege to spontaneously explosive cries for power in the experience of its absence.[3] In either case, they represent a world of human action considerably wider than the restrictive parameters of psychiatric reality.

*Suggesting Something "Better": Viewing Dangerousness*
*within Its Sociopolitical Context*

Having stated what I think is wrong with psychiatric predictions, let me make a suggestion for something "imperfectly" better. We have argued that decisions about who needs to be confined in maximum security are inherently political. Hence, if these decisions must be made (as they will be in the foreseeable future), they should be rendered in a more explicitly political form, such as that of a jury hearing before one's "peers." We have also argued that psychiatric predictions are not particularly expert in sorting out dangerous persons or psychopathic individuals. They are expert only in the careful management of their users' professional identities. These careful management practices should be discarded, and the work of psychiatric professionals should be displayed but one input within the context of advocacy and cross-examination. If this is done, the usefulness of psychiatric judgments can be preserved, without treating these judgments as the objective products of expert technologies. Psychiatric professionals can be quizzed as to the basis for their opinions. Decision-makers can be exposed to their inferential logic-in-use as well as their justificatory logic of professional reconstruction.

The suggestion of a juried hearing is based upon observations of several of the few cases in which Lima State patients appealed the recommendations set forth by psychiatric review teams. Legal advocates debated the issue of a patient's dangerousness and/or need for confinement and interrogated the "experts" involved in a decision. In one case, the psychiatric team had concluded that a patient was "a creature of pure impulse, with no controls whatsoever, no conscience, and no feelings of remorse or sensibility" and that he was "considered to be immediately dangerous to others and in continued need of hospitalization in a maximum-security facility." During the hearing, legal advocates produced evidence that the patient "had not shown aggressiveness or assaultiveness" during his stay at the hospital. Testimony by hospital staff indicated "that the patient could be adequately cared for outside a maximum-security institution." In light of this additional evidence, the court reversed the recommendation of the "experts" and decided that the patient did not need maximum security. The court was informed by more than psychiatric predictions. It should be. As such, we conclude that the professional prediction of dangerousness should be replaced by public adjudication. This would ensure that judgments regarding involuntary confinement remain within the explicitly political arena to which they belong.

The institutionalization of mandatory adjudication may function to "de-expertise" the opinions of psychiatric decision-makers. This may (and in all likelihood will) elicit considerable opposition from psychiatric professionals themselves. According to Brodsky, the well-versed cross-examiner can be "an expert witness' nightmare." While a system of advocacy "provides a base of common challenge points, it may, for the uncertain witness, precipitate a bad experience."[4] Nonetheless, our consistent discovery of inconsistency, disguised uncertainty, and negotiated objectivity suggests that public adjudication is necessary. The appearance of expert decision-making should not be allowed to replace the "reality" of political judgment.

**Concluding Remarks**

In this book I have attended to the problem of what psychiatric professionals actually do in diagnosing the disturbances and troubles of others. It has been discovered that diagnosticians do a lot of things that directly affect decisions about patients, but which may have little to do with patients' own troubles in everyday life. I have catalogued what diagnosticians do in terms of a number of essential and contingent features of their social interaction with each other. Through the use of excerpts from diagnosticians' own conversations and reports I have tried to display my own basis for claiming a certain knowledge about what they do and how they do it. In completing my analysis, I have suggested that this study theoretically supports a social reaction perspective on deviance. Pragmatically, it suggests that psychiatric opinions are essentially political judgments and should be "deexpertised" through a system of public advocacy and adjudication.

Throughout this report I have been concerned with the practices through which "expert psychiatric knowledge" is accomplished and "expert status" afforded its creators. In concluding this report, I have formulated certain moral and political reservations about relatively unrestrained displays of psychiatric expertise. These reservations are supported by the data, which suggest that expert psychiatric knowledge is a well-managed "appearance of objectivity" rather than a set of "objective facts." Its "factualness" should not be taken for granted. It counts and counts heavily in the lives of patients whose psychiatric realities are diagnosed.

Because of the serious consequences of psychiatric decision-making, I believe that the basis for its "factualness," its dependence on a process of negotiated social interaction, should be displayed for public scrutiny. We hope that the presentation of our findings represents a step in this direction. We are confident that the public adjudication of each attempt to confine someone as dangerous or in need of maximum security will represent another more permanent step. The implementation of this step should actualize the spirit of Judge David Bazelon's ruling in the case of *Covington* v. *Cameron*.[5] That decision stated that it was the responsibility of the court to see that psychiatric decision-makers reach "reasoned" and not "unreasonable" conclusions, employ "proper criteria," and "do not overlook anything of substantial relevance." To bring decision-makers out of enclaves of expertise and into the public scrutiny of the courtroom should advance these goals. I thus conclude by agreeing with Judge Bazelon that "to do less would abandon the interests affected to the absolute power of administrative officials."[6]

### Notes

1. Abraham Kaplan, *The Conduct of Inquiry: Methodology for the Behavioral Sciences* (Scranton, Pa.: Chandler Publishing Co., 1964).

2. The suggestion that human conduct is intricately related to, rather than determined by, the socioeconomic forces which shape the fate of collectivities is quite deliberate. We are here presenting a "critical analysis" which envisions individual actions as restrained, but not caused, by infrastructural variables. For a more detailed discussion of the reified individuality of the criminal law, see Barry Krisberg, *Crime and Privilege* (Englewood Cliffs, N.J.: Prentice-Hall, 1975). Krisberg makes the important distinction between equality based upon "formal rationality" (or individual justice) and that based upon "substantive rationality" (or social justice). It is the former which is expanded by the present criminal justice system. As Krisberg points out, however, the problem is that "the poor and those who are denied the benefits of privilege, are not served by the 'equal' system of justice. Their demands that the law administer the equalization of economic and social privilege is blocked by judges and administrators who proclaim that the requirements of formal, rational law prohibit special favors" (p. 49).

3. There is no attempt here to romanticize "proletarian violence." The relation between the meaning of violence for the actor and the experience of relative powerlessness has been mapped out in numerous investigations. Cf. Lynn Curtis, *Violence, Race, and Culture* (Lexington, Mass.: Lexington Books, 1975).

4. Stanley L. Brodsky, *Psychologists in the Criminal Justice System* (Carbondale, Illinois: Admark, 1972), p. 95.

5. Cf. *Covington* v. *Cameron*, 419 F.2d 617 (D.C. cir. 1969).

6. Bazelon is here excerpted in Jonas Robitscher, "The Right to Treatment: A Social-Legal Approach to the Plight of the State Hospital Patient," *Villanova Law Review* 18 (November 1972): 19.

# Bibliography

Ash, P.

    1949. The reliability of psychiatric diagnosis. *Journal of Abnormal and Social Psychology* 44: 272-276.

Balint, Michael.

    1957. *The Doctor, His Patient and the Illness.* New York: International Press.

Baxter, Seymour; Chodorkoff, Bernard; and Underhill, Robert.

    1968. Psychiatric emergencies: dispositional determinants and the validity of the decision to admit. *American Journal of Psychiatry* 124 (May): 100-104.

Beck, A.T.; Ward, C.H.; Mendelson, M.; Mock, J.E.; and Erbaugh, J.K.

    1962. Reliability of psychiatric diagnosis: a study of consistency of clinical judgments and ratings. *American Journal of Psychiatry* 119 (October): 351-357.

Becker, Howard S.

    1963. *Outsiders: Studies in the Sociology of Deviance.* New York: The Free Press.

    1973. Labelling theory reconsidered, in H. Becker, ed., *Outsiders: Studies in the Sociology of Deviance.* New York: The Free Press.

Bem, D.J.

    1970. *Beliefs, Attitudes and Human Affairs.* Belmont, California: Brooks-Cole.

Berger, Peter, and Luckmann, Thomas.

    1966. *The Social Construction of Reality.* New York: Anchor Books.

Bittner, Egon.

    1967. Police discretion in apprehending the mentally ill. *Social Problems* 14 (Winter): 278-292.

    1969. The police on skid-row: a study of peace keeping. *American Sociological Review* 32: 669-715.

Blum, Alan F.

    1970. The sociology of mental illness, in J. Douglas, ed., *Deviance and Respectability.* New York: Basic Books.

Brodsky, Stanley L.

    1972. *Psychologists in the Criminal Justice System.* Carbondale, Illinois: Admark.

Buckner, H. Taylor.

    1971. *Deviance, Reality and Change.* New York: Random House.

Caulfield, James M.

    1974. Ohio commitments of the mentally ill offender. *Capital University Law Review* 4, 1: 1-36.

233

234

Cicourel, Aaron V.

1964. *Method and Measurement in Sociology*. New York: The Free Press.

1970*a*. Basic and normative rules in the negotiation of status and role, in H. Dreitzel, ed., *Recent Sociology No. 2*. New York: Macmillan.

1970*b*. The acquisition of social structure: toward a developmental sociology of language and meaning, in J. Douglas, ed., *Understanding Everyday Life*. Chicago: Aldine.

1974. *Cognitive Sociology: Language and Meaning in Social Interaction*. New York: The Free Press.

., and Kituse, John J.

1963. A note on the use of official statistics. *Social Problems* 11: 139-159.

Coulter, Jeff.

1975. *The Operations of Mental Health Personnel in an Urban Area*. Manchester, England: University of Manchester, unpublished dissertation.

Curtis, Lynn.

1975. *Violence, Race and Culture*. Lexington, Massachusetts: Lexington Books.

Daniels, Arelene Kaplan.

1970. The social construction of psychiatric diagnoses, in H. Dreitzel, ed., *Recent Sociology No. 2*. New York: Macmillan.

Denzin, Norman K.

1970. *The Research Act in Sociology: A Theoretical Introduction to Sociological Methods*. London: Butterworths.

Dershowitz, A.

1969. Psychiatrists' power in civil commitment. *Psychology Today* 2 (February): 43-47.

Dohrenwend, Bruce and Barbara.

1969. *Social Status and Psychiatric Disorder*. New York: John Wiley.

Douglas, Jack.

1970. *Understanding Everyday Life: Toward a Reconstruction of Sociological Knowledge*. Chicago: Aldine.

Dreitzel, Hans Peter.

1970. *Recent Sociology No. 2: Patterns of Communicative Behavior*. New York: Macmillan.

Emerson, Richard.

1962. Power and dependence relations. *American Sociological Review* 27 (February): 31-41.

Fisher, Joel.

1969. Negroes and whites and rates of mental illness: reconsideration of a myth. *Psychiatry* 32 (November): 428-446.

Franks, David D.

1976. Social power, role-taking and the structure of imperceptiveness:

toward a redefinition of false consciousness. *Annals of Phenomeno-logical Sociology* 1: 93-111.

Freudenberg, R.K., and Robertson, J.P.
1956. Symptoms in relation to psychiatric diagnosis and treatment. *A.M.A. Archives of Neurological Psychiatry* 76: 14-22.

Garfinkel, Harold.
1967. *Studies in Ethnomethodology.* Englewood Cliffs, N.J.: Prentice-Hall.
1972. Common sense knowledge of social structures: the documentary method of interpretation, in J. Manis and B. Meltzer, eds., *Symbolic Interaction.* Boston: Allyn and Bacon.

Gibbs, Jack P.
1972. Issues in defining deviant behavior, in Robert A. Scott and Jack D. Douglas, eds., *Theoretical Perspectives on Deviance.* New York: Basic Books.

Giddens, Anthony.
1977. *The New Rules of the Sociological Method: A Positive Critique of Interpretive Sociology.* New York: Basic Books.

Goffman, Erving.
1962. *Asylums.* Chicago: Aldine Publishing Company.
1971. *Relations in Public.* Garden City, New York: Doubleday.
1974. *Frame Analysis.* New York: Harper and Row.

Gorgoff, Norman N.
1974. Simulation and social research: incarceration and subjective mean-ing. A paper presented at the 1974 meeting of the American Socio-logical Association, Montreal.

Gottheil, E.; Kramer, M.; and Huruich, M.S.
1966. Intake procedures and psychiatric decisions. *Comprehensive Psychiatry* 7: 207-215.

Gouldner, Alvin.
1968. The sociologist as partisan: sociology and the welfare state. *American Sociological Review* 3 (May): 103-116.

Gove, Walter R.
1970. Societal reaction as an explanation of mental illness: an evaluation. *American Sociological Review* 35 (October): 873-874.
1975a. *The Labelling Theory of Deviance: Evaluating a Perspective.* New York: Halstead Press.
1975b. The labelling theory of mental illness: a reply to Scheff. *American Sociological Review* 40 (April): 242-247.
———., and Fain, Terry.
1973. The stigma of mental hospitalization: an attempt to evaluate its consequences. *Archives of General Psychiatry* 28 (April): 494-500.
———., and Howell, Patrick.
1974. Individual resources and mental hospitalization: a comparison and

evaluating of the social reaction and psychiatric perspectiveness. *American Sociological Review* 39 (February): 86-100.

————., and Tutor, Jeanette.

    1973. Adult sex roles and mental illness. *American Journal of Sociology* 78 (January): 812-835.

Greenley, James R.

    1972. The psychiatric patient's family and length of hospitalization. *Journal of Health and Social Behavior* 13 (March): 25-37.

Halleck, Seymour L.

    1971. *The Politics of Therapy.* New York: Harper and Row.

Hammer, Muriel.

    1963. Influence of small social networks of factors on mental hospitalization. *Human Organizations* 22 (Winter): 243-251.

Heider, Fritz.

    1958. *The Psychology of Interpersonal Relations.* New York: Wiley.

Hyman, Herbert.

    1954. *Interviewing in Social Research.* Chicago: University of Chicago Press.

Kaplan, Abraham.

    1964. *The Conduct of Inquiry: Methodology for the Behavioral Sciences.* Scranton, Pennsylvania: Chandler Publishing Co.

Katz, M.M.; Cole, J.O.; and Lowery, H.A.

    1964. Nonspecificity of diagnosis of paranoid schizophrenia. *Archives of General Psychiatry* 11: 197-202.

Kirk, Stuart.

    1974. The impact of labelling on rejection of the mentally ill: an experimental study. *Journal of Health and Social Behavior* 15 (June): 108-117.

Kituse, John I.

    1962. Societal reaction to deviant behavior: problems of theory and method. *Social Problems* 9: 247-256.

    1975. The "new conception of deviance" and its critics, in Walter Gove, ed., *The Labelling of Deviance: Evaluating a Perspective.* New York: Halstead Press.

————., and Spector, Malcolm.

    1975. Deviance and social problems: some parallel issues. *Social Problems* 23 (Fall).

Kozol, H.R.; Boucher, R.; and Garofalo, R.

    1972. The diagnosis and treatment of dangerousness. *Crime and Delinquency* 8 (October): 371-392.

Krisberg, Berry.

    1975. *Crime and Privilege: Toward a New Criminology.* Englewood Cliffs, New Jersey: Prentice-Hall.

Laing, R.D., and Esterson, A.
  1964. *Sanity, Madness and the Family.* Baltimore, Maryland: Ballantine
    Books.
Lemert, Edwin M.
  1951. *Social Pathology.* New York: McGraw-Hill.
  1972. *Human Deviance, Social Problems and Social Control.* Englewood
    Cliffs, New Jersey: Prentice-Hall.
Linsky, Arnold S.
  1970. Community homogeneity and exclusion of the mentally ill: rejec-
    tion v. consensus about deviance. *Journal of Health and Social
    Behavior* 14 (December): 304-311.
Lofland, John.
  1969. *Deviance and Identity.* Englewood Cliffs, N.J.: Prentice-Hall.
  1971. *Analyzing Social Setting: A Guide to Qualitative Observation and
    Analysis.* Belmont, California: Wadsworth Publishing Company.
Manning, Peter K.
  1970. Talking and becoming: a view of organizational socialization, in
    J. Douglas, ed., *Understanding Everyday Life.* Chicago: Aldine.
Maryl, William.
  1973. Ethnomethodology: sociology without society. *Catalyst* 7 (Winter):
    15-28.
McDermott, J.F.; Harrison, S.I.; Schrager, P.W.; Killins, E.; Lindy, J.; and
Waggoner, R.W.
  1967. Social class and mental illness in children: the diagnosis of organity
    and mental retardation. *Journal of the American Academy of Child
    Psychiatry* 6: 309-320.
Mead, George Herbert.
  1918. The psychology of punitive justice. *American Journal of Sociology*
    23: 577-602.
  1932. *Mind, Self and Society.* Chicago: University of Chicago Press.
Megargee, E.
  1970. The prediction of violence with psychological tests, in C. Speilber-
    ger, ed., *Current Topics in Clinical and Community Psychology.*
    New York: The Academic Press.
Mehan, Hugh, and Woods, Houston.
  1975. *The Reality of Ethnomethodology.* New York: John Wiley.
Mehlman, B.
  1952. The reliability of psychiatric diagnosis. *Journal of Abnormal and
    Social Psychology* 47: 577-578.
Miller, Dorthy, and Schwartz, Michael.
  1966. County lunacy commission hearings: some observations of commit-
    ments to a state mental hospital. *Social Problems* 14 (Summer):
    26-35.

Mishler, Elliot, and Wexler, Nancy.
    1963. Decision processes in psychiatric hospitalization. *American Sociological Review* 28 (August): 576-587.

Monahan, John.
    1975. The prediction of dangerousness, in D. Chappell and J. Monahan, eds., *Violence and Criminal Justice.* Lexington, Mass.: D.C. Heath and Co.

Norris, V.
    1959. *Mental Illness in London, Maudsley Monographs No. 6.* London: Chapman and Hall.

Pasamanick, Benjamin; Dinitz, Simon; and Lefton, Mark.
    1959. Psychiatric orientation and its relation to diagnosis and treatment in a mental hospital. *American Journal of Psychiatry* 116: 127-132.

Pasamanick, Benjamin; Dinitz, Simon; and Scarpitti, Frank.
    1967. *Schizophrenics in the Community.* New York: Appleton-Century-Crofts.

Perinbanayagam, R.S.
    1974. The definition of the situation: an analysis of the ethnomethodology and dramaturgical view. *The Sociological Quarterly* 15 (August): 521-541.

Perrucci, Robert.
    1974. *Circle of Madness: Being Insane and Institutionalized in America.* Englewood Cliffs, N.J.: Prentice-Hall.

Pfohl, Stephen J.
    1975*a. Right to Treatment Litigation: A Consideration of Judicial Intervention into Mental Health Policy.* Columbus, Ohio: Ohio Division of Mental Health.
    1975*b.* Social role analysis: the ethnomethodological critique. *Sociology and Social Research* 59, 3 (April): 343-265.

Phillips, Derek L.
    1963. Rejection: a possible consequence of seeking help for mental disorders. *American Sociological Review* 28: 963-972.

Phillips, Leslie, and Draguns, Juris G.
    1971. "Classification of the behavioral disorders." *Annual Review of Psychology*, 22: 447-482.

Pollner, Melvin.
    1974. Sociological and common-sense models of the labelling process, in Roy Turner, ed., *Ethnomethodology: Selected Readings.* Middlesex, England: Penguin Books.

Prus, Robert C.
    1974. Resisting designations: an extension of attribution theory into a negotiated context. *Sociological Inquiry* 45, 1: 3-14.
    1975. Labelling theory: a reconceptualization and a propositional

statement on typing. *Sociological Focus* 8, 1 (January): 79-96.
Rappaport, Maurice.
    1973. Selective drug utilization in the management of psychoses. Paper read at Western Psychological Association Meeting, April 1973. Abstracted in *Psychology Today* 8 (November): 39, 138.
Raven, B.H.
    1965. Social influence and power, in I.D. Stein and M. Fishbein, eds., *Current Studies in Social Psychology*. New York: Holt, Rinehart and Winston.
Robitscher, Jonas.
    1972. The right to treatment: a socio-legal approach to the plight of the state hospital patient. *Villanova Law Review* 18,1 (November): 11-32.
Rosenhan, David L.
    1973. On being sane in insane places. *Science* 179 (January): 250-258.
Sampson, Harold; Messinger, Sheldon; and Towne, Robert D.
    1962. Family processes and becoming a mental patient. *American Journal of Sociology* 68: 88-96.
Scheff, Thomas J.
    1964. The social reaction to deviance: ascriptive elements in the psychiatric screening of mental patients in a midwestern state. *Social Problems* 11 (Spring): 401-413.
    1966. *Being Mentally Ill: A Sociological Theory*. Chicago: Aldine.
    1967. *Mental Illness and the Social Processes*. New York: Harper and Row.
    1968. Negotiating reality: notes on power in the assessment of responsibility. *Social Problems* 16, 1 (September): 3-17.
    1974. The labelling theory of mental illness. *American Sociological Review* 30 (June): 444-452.
    1975. Reply to Chauncey and Gove. *American Sociological Review* 40, 2 (April): 252-257.
Schegloff, Emmanuel A.
    1972. Notes on a conversational practice: formulating place, in David Sudnow, ed., *Studies in Social Interaction*. New York: The Free Press.
Schmidt, H.O., Fonda, C.P.
    1956. The reliability of psychiatric diagnosis: a new look. *Journal of Abnormal and Social Psychology* 52: 262-267.
Schultz, Alfred.
    1971. *Collected Papers II: Studies in Social Theory*. The Hague: Martinus Nijhoff.
Schultz, Alfred, and Luckmann, Thomas.
    1973. *The Structures of the Life-World*. Evanston, Illinois: Northwestern University Press.

Shader, R.I.; Binstock, W.A.; Orly, J.I.; and Scott, D.
    1969. "Biasing factors in diagnosis and disposition. *Comprehensive Psychiatry* 10: 81-89.

Shorer, C.E.
    1968. Mistakes in the diagnosis of schizophrenia. *American Journal of Psychiatry* 124: 1057-1062.

Smart, Barry.
    1976. *Sociology, Phenomenology and Marxian Analysis.* London: Routledge and Kegan Paul.

Spitzer, S., and Denzin, N.
    1968. *The Mental Patient: Studies in the Sociology of Deviance.* New York: McGraw-Hill Book Company.

Stanford, Phil.
    1972. Model "clockwork orange" prison—patuxent institute for defective delinquents. *New York Times Magazine* (September 17, 1972).

Steadman, Henry, and Cocozza, J.
    1974. *Careers of the Criminally Insane: Excessive Social Control of Deviance.* Lexington, Massachusetts: Lexington Books.

Stone, Alan A.
    1975. *Mental Health and Law: A System in Transition.* Rockville, Maryland: National Institute of Mental Health.

Szasz, Thomas.
    1968. The myth of mental illness, in S. Spitzer and N. Danzin, eds., *The Mental Patient: Studies in the Sociology of Deviance.* New York: McGraw-Hill Book Co.

Tannenbaum, Frank.
    1951. *Crime and the Community.* New York: McGraw-Hill Book Co.

Temerlin, Maurice K.
    1968. Suggestion effects in psychiatric diagnosis. *Journal of Mental Disease* 147 (April): 349-353.

Ullmann, Leonard D., and Krasner, Leonard.
    1969. *A Psychological Approach to Abnormal Behavior.* Englewood Cliffs, N.J.: Prentice-Hall.

Wegner, Dennis R., and Fletcher, C. Richard.
    1969. The effect of legal counsel on admissions to a state hospital: a confrontation of professions. *Journal of Health and Social Behavior* 10 (June): 349-353.

Wenk, E.; Robinson, J.; and Smith, G.
    1972. Can violence be predicted? *Crime and Delinquency*, 18 393-402.

Wilde, William A.
    1968. Decision-making in a psychiatric screening agency. *Journal of Health and Social Behavior* 9 (September): 215-221.

Wilkinson, Greg S.
    1974. Psychiatric disorder dramaturgically considered. *Sociological Quarterly* 15, 1 (Winter): 143-158.
Yarrow, Marion; Schwartz, Charlotte; Murphy, Harriet; and Deasy, Leila.
    1955. The psychological meaning of mental illness in the family. *Journal of Social Issues* 11, 4: 12-24.
Zigler, E., and Philips, L.
    1961. Psychiatric diagnosis and symptomatology. *Journal of Abnormal and Social Psychology* 63: 69-75.
Ziskin, Jay.
    1970. *Coping with Psychiatric and Psychological Testimony.* Beverly Hills, Cal.: Law and Psychology Press.
Zubin, Joseph.
    1967. Classification of the behavioral disorders, *Annual Review of Psychology* 18: 373-406.
    1969. Cross-national study of diagnosis of the mental disorders: methodology and planning. *American Journal of Psychiatry* 125, 19 (April supplement): 12-20.
————., Eron, L.D.; and Schumer, F.
    1965. *Experimental Approaches to Assessment of Behavior in Psychopathology.* New York: Wiley.

# Name Index

# Name Index

# Subject Index

# Subject Index

Patients' self-presentation, 154–166
Previewing the patient, 127–135, 217
Psychiatric decision-making: adequacy
    of, 15–16; and dangerousness,
    18–20, 22; interactional work
    of, 22–26; modifications of,
    228–229; politics of, 226–
    228; sociological accounts
    of, 20–22; unreliability of,
    16–17, 224–226; validity of,
    17–18, 224–226
Psychiatric diagnosis: agents of, 49;
    anticipation consequences of,
    206–208; de-socializing troubles
    through, 208–212; social class
    and, 22, 36–37, 39, 208–212;
    work of, 49–50
Psychiatric expertise: appearance of,
    93–98; critiques of, 15–22; faith
    in, 5; language of, 218; produc-
    tion of 212–213
Psychiatric interviewing: cognitive
    style, 137–142; substantive
    themes, 142–152
Psychiatric records: consequences of
    using, 131–135, 217; and diag-
    nosis, 127–135; reflexive use of,
    129–130
Psychiatric team members: disciplinary
    differences, 152–154; formal
    preparation, 85–86; as imputa-
    tional specialists, 3–4, 49;
    initial involvement, 84; past
    experience, 85; professional
    orientation, 84–85; purposes-
    at-hand, 93–98

Psychopathic offenders: assumptions
    about, 111–119; legal issues,
    88–89
Purposes-at-hand: appearing expert,
    94–98; making sense of patients,
    93–94; multiple purposes, 93–
    94; and psychiatric decisions,
    220–221

Reconciliatory logic, 180–189, 218
Reflexivity: and ethnomethodology,
    45–46; and psychiatric record
    reading, 130–131; unnoticed,
    46, 221

Selective hearing, 148–152, 218
Selective questioning, 143–146, 218
Social control: and dangerousness,
    3–4; and psychiatric individua-
    tion, 226–228
Social power: and ethnomethodology,
    52–54, 224; and psychiatric
    decisions, 189–191, 203–206,
    219
Social status: consequences of, 219;
    negotiating, 189–203. *See also*
    Social power
Societal reaction perspective: debate
    over, 34–44; and ethnomethod-
    ology, 44–47, 222–224; and
    labeling theory, 32–34; support
    for, 223; as a theoretical frame-
    work, 6–7, 31–32

Triangulation, 63–64

# About the Author

**Stephen J. Pfohl** is an assistant professor of sociology at Boston College. He received the B.A. from the Catholic University of America and the M.A. and Ph.D. from Ohio State University. He has been involved in research on health service delivery for migrant farm workers, served as a full-time research consultant for the Ohio Division of Mental Health, and as an assistant to the editor of the *Journal of Research in Crime and Delinquency*, and has recently participated in the court-ordered reclassification of all inmates in the Alabama correctional system. His recent publications have focused on child abuse, criminal violence, ethnomethodology, predictions of dangerousness, and the implications of right to treatment litigation. He is currently collaborating on a project investigating the relationship between the social structure of dating and the crime of rape. He is also completing a book, *Deviance and Social Control*, for publication with D.C. Heath.